Yogic Management of
Common Diseases

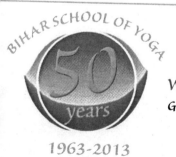

BIHAR SCHOOL OF YOGA

50 years

1963-2013
GOLDEN JUBILEE

WORLD YOGA CONVENTION 2013
GANGA DARSHAN, MUNGER, BIHAR, INDIA
23rd-27th October 2013

Yogic Management of Common Diseases

Dr Swami Karmananda
MBBS (Sydney)

Under the Guidance of
Swami Satyananda Saraswati

Yoga Publications Trust, Munger, Bihar, India

Published by Bihar School of Yoga
    First edition 1983
    Reprinted 1986, 1992

Published by Yoga Publications Trust
    Reprinted 2001, 2003, 2005, 2006, 2008
    Second edition 2010
    Reprinted 2013

ISBN: 978-81-85787-24-4

Publisher and distributor: Yoga Publications Trust, Ganga Darshan, Munger, Bihar, India.

Website: www.biharyoga.net
         www.rikhiapeeth.net

Printed at Thomson Press (India) Limited, New Delhi, 110001

Man today is sick because he thinks he is sick. Sickness and disease have no place in the life of a person who does not accept and tolerate the self-limiting thoughts which are the real seeds of our myriad ailments. We stand hypnotized by the belief that disease and illness are our fate and destiny, rather than health and bliss, which are truly our birthright and heritage. In order to emerge from our mass hypnosis and collective hysteria and to experience health, joy and creative fulfilment, we must make a systematic application of yoga in our daily lives.

—*Swami Satyananda Saraswati*

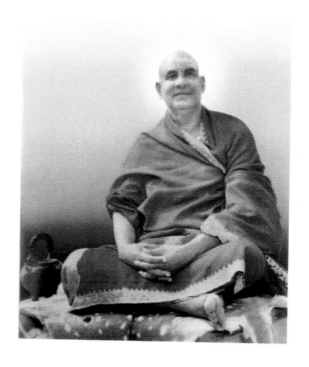

Dedication

In humility we offer this dedication to
Swami Sivananda Saraswati, who initiated
Swami Satyananda Saraswati into the secrets of yoga.

Contents

x

Introduction

The *Yogic Management of Common Diseases* is a series of short essays on the common diseases which plague humanity. The range of topics covers the majority of mild chronic diseases which are most amenable to yogic therapy.

Each essay is designed to highlight certain key points of the disease in question so that the reader, whether a doctor, therapist, healer, yoga practitioner, patient or interested layperson, can perceive the overall clinical picture and gain understanding of the physical, emotional, mental and psychic factors underlying its cause from the yogic point of view. The yogic path to freedom from each condition is given at the end of each chapter.

The aim of this book

This book is intended to inspire people to practise yoga and to raise themselves out of their condition, which seems to surround them like an impenetrable and inescapable wall. It aims to inform people that a way out exists. It is this very information which is so important, for it carries energy and becomes the idea in the mind which, when put into practice, becomes the vehicle for the cessation of their suffering. It is also intended as a guide to doctors and therapists seeking new alternatives and indicates to them the broad range of yogic practices applicable for conditions which have, until now, not proven amenable to conventional medical therapies.

1

Many diseases have been left out of this book because they do not fall into the category of 'common' and, no doubt, these will be included in a full textbook on yoga therapy. It is also not our intention to give all the details of the diseases discussed in this book. Doctors and therapists already know the anatomy, physiology and pathology of these simple problems and to include these aspects would necessitate a volume far beyond a book of this kind. The interested layperson should consult the relevant medical reference texts for fuller information, if so desired.

The necessity of a guru

We cannot emphasize strongly enough that all therapy should be undertaken only under expert guidance and not just from books or inexperienced practitioners. At the same time, therapy that has been undertaken with a half-hearted attitude, with irregular practice and a distracted mind is worse than useless, for the practitioner usually ends up blaming yoga for his or her own failure. When the practices are taught and learnt correctly, the practitioner must at least halt the progressive deterioration of his condition and gain some degree of improvement, if not total freedom from disease.

Much depends on the degree of severity of the disease and its duration. There can be no doubt that yoga is much more effective when applied to a newly occurring condition in a young person than when undertaken as a last resort because all other methods have failed. In this regard it is up to the therapist, in conjunction with an empathetic medical practitioner, to choose those techniques from the long list at the end of each chapter which suit the individual's needs and which solve the inevitable difficulties which arise as the cure progresses. The teacher is necessary, for he or she can recognize these difficulties as they come up and before they give rise to another disease which may be more difficult to cure than the first. It should be noted that it is always dangerous to treat yourself.

Yoga and medicine

It is essential that before undertaking yoga therapy a full medical examination be performed by a qualified practitioner. This is imperative in order to:

1. Ascertain the exact nature of the condition.
2. Find out whether there are complications. For example, if someone with diabetes also has high blood pressure, the programme of yogic treatment will be quite different from that of the diabetic with no complications.
3. Decide whether yogic or medical treatment should be the first line of approach. Many inexperienced therapists jump in with yoga when medical therapy would prove the faster and more efficient means to a cure, and vice versa. This is the typical one-sided approach of a closed and narrow mind.

Only a qualified professional in the healing or medical world can decide whether a disease can be treated by their particular discipline.

Anyone who has experience in yoga therapy will that a guru or qualified teacher is vital. For example, it is often necessary to continue medical treatment for some time before the yogic practices are established and working effectively. Only an experienced individual or doctor can indicate when medicines can be reduced and yoga practices relied on for the maintenance of health. The teacher instructs the patient in preparatory practices for the yoga techniques specified for each individual condition.

Though yoga and medicine work hand in hand to safely re-establish health, only yoga can truly bring about and maitain health, for yoga views life and disease in a revolutionary light. Instead of seeing disease as something to be feared and quickly eradicated, yoga teaches us that, from a spiritual point of view, disease is our teacher and friend.

Disease indicates that we have been making an error in our lifestyle or thinking and have become unbalanced. It shows us that we must make some changes if we are to live a healthier, fuller and more joyous existence. Yoga teaches us that we must learn to use and value our sufferings as springboards in our spiritual evolution. Somehow we have lost our awareness of who we are and how we can lead useful and aware lives. Loss of awareness allows disease to creep in. When we are sick, we are forced by nature to wake up to our transgressions of natural laws. Regaining our awareness through yogic practices is the key to health. The yogic process brings about rebalance, insight, understanding and appreciation of the universal, natural laws which operate in the world we live in.

Ashram life
One of the most powerful and useful aspects of yogic therapy is ashram life. For the sincere individual who really wishes to regain positive physical and mental health, and insight into the fundamental errors of lifestyle and thinking which have led to disease, a short stay in an ashram is a shortcut to learning a new and healthy lifestyle and offers one of the most intense exposures to yoga.

Any therapy undertaken in the positive atmosphere of the ashram is supercharged with pranic, vital energy and supported by the glowing, cheerful health of the inmates who are living examples of what yoga allows us to achieve.

Yogic therapy involves all aspects of ashram life, both formal and informal. Formal training in asanas, pranayama, cleansing practices, meditation and yoga nidra forms the basic therapeutic program. Equally beneficial, however, is the informal exposure to the practices of satsang, karma yoga perhaps in the form of structured, light work within the ashram and bhakti yoga, usually in the form of nada yoga, the chanting of mantras and kirtan at night. The natural, relaxed atmosphere of ashram life provides an ideal setting for emotional and physical renewal.

In Ganga Darshan ashram at Bihar School of Yoga, Munger, Bihar, India, we have seen time and again that when individuals come for therapy they are amazed at how easy and simple yogic therapy can be. They quickly begin to feel recharged and revitalized and soon appreciate that there is another and better way of approaching their bodies, attitudes and ways of relating to the world. When these people return home and place the simple, powerful and effective ashram principles within the framework of their daily lives, dramatic changes take place far beyond what most people dreamed possible. The human organism realigns and becomes harmonized to natural cycles and energies. Changes take place beneath the purely intellectual or conscious mind, within the powerful subconscious and intuitive spaces dormant in all of us. We feel good, even if we do not consciously understand exactly why.

Beyond yoga therapy

After yoga therapy has been instituted and practised for some time, it becomes easier, in retrospect, to see what has happened. Even if we leave the yoga practices when a cure has taken place, the memories and impressions remain and eventually we realize that yoga transcends the purely therapeutic approach to disease, and we begin to see it as a valuable aid to healthy living and spiritual evolution.

Further reading

All the practices of yoga suggested in the *Yogic Management of Common Diseases* are fully described and illustrated in the two basic and complete yogic textbooks, *Asana Pranayama Mudra Bandha* and *Meditations from the Tantras*, both by Swami Satyananda Saraswati and published by the Yoga Publications Trust. These textbooks provide a basis for both therapist and patient, describing the practices, explaining their benefits and contraindications and acting as reference guides for future yogic development.

Other books in the therapy line published by Yoga Publications Trust are: *Yoga and Cardiovascular Management, The Effects of Yoga on Hypertension, Yogic Management of Asthma and Diabetes, The Practices of Yoga for the Digestive System,*

Exploring Yoga and Cancer and *Yogic Management of Cancer.* These books give fuller descriptions of the body system involved, the disease process and the use of yogic therapy in combination with other systems.

Texts such as *Teachings of Swami Satyananda, Yoga from Shore to Shore, Sure Ways to Self-Realization, Hatha Yoga Pradipika*, and the other Yoga Publications Trust publications put yoga therapy into perspective and give a broad view of the application of yoga to healthy living and high thinking. They are the basis for the total regeneration and transformation of the individual from a purely sensual life and its enjoyments, with its inherent diseases and suffering, to a spiritual and yogic based life which leads us to health, joy and eventually self-realization.

The Yoga Research Foundation, established by Swami Satyananda Saraswati at Ganga Darshan Ashram, Munger, Bihar, in 1984, has an extensive collection of books dealing specifically with yoga as a healing system. One of the main aims of the foundation is to act as a focal point, inspiring and correlating international research on this and related topics. Facilities are also being established for independent investigations into the effects of yogic and tantric techniques on both physiological and psychological levels, with the help of qualified doctors and scientists from the international community. As the research is centred within the ashram, opportunity is also given for dealing more deeply with both exoteric and esoteric practices, moving from basic issues of sickness and health to realization of our potential faculties and inner nature.

Head and Neck

Short- and Long-Sightedness

"The eyes are the mirror of the soul and reveal much of our essential nature. At the same time, vision is our most precious sense. We rely on the eyes for a large percentage of our information about the outside world and our understanding of life." The phrase "Do you see what I mean?" implies that a large part of our mental functioning relies on the visual sense. At the same time it has been reported by yogis that they do not need the eyes to see, being able to know in detail, through the higher strata of consciousness, of events which take place at great distances from their physical bodies. Vision is indeed a mysterious thing.

Structure of the eye

The eye is the only part of the brain which projects outside the cranium, the bony box which protects the brain. The white area of the eye is called sclera. This becomes transparent centrally and is called the cornea. Behind the cornea is the iris, which gives the eye its characteristic colour. The centre of the iris is a hole, called the pupil, which allows light into the eye. The iris constantly contracts and dilates in order to adjust the amount of light coming into the eye. Behind the cornea is the lens which adjusts our vision to distance. The inside of the eye is filled with fluid.

Light passes through the lens and falls on the inner back wall of the eye, which is called the retina. The retina

9

has specialized sensory receptors called rods and cones, which react to shading, black and white, and colour. The images projected onto the retina pass via the optic nerves to the back (occipital) part of the cerebrum of the brain. The cerebrum integrates the images coming from both eyes. Because we have binocular vision, two eyes focusing on an object, we can appreciate depth and distance, size and spatial relationships. More and more we see that vision is indeed a miracle of creation.

Short- and long-sightedness

The lens is situated in the centre of the eye and is responsible for the bending of incoming rays of light so that they converge onto the retina and thereby stimulate nerve cells to produce a clear and accurate picture of the image being viewed. The process of bending light is called refraction. If the lens fails to focus light exactly onto the retina, the picture is blurred and this is called refractive error. This may also occur because the shape of the eye distorts from a near perfect sphere, either elongating or shortening. The following refractive errors are the most common:

1. *Myopia* (short-sightedness), in which the lens is too thick and the image falls short of the retina, resulting in an inability to focus on distant objects. This is most common in young people.
2. *Hypermetropia* (long-sightedness), which is the opposite of myopia. It is more common in old age.
3. *Astigmatism*, which is caused by variations and unevenness in the lens.

These distortions of eye function are so common today that we fail to even think of them as correctable by means other than glasses. Our hair falls out, teeth have to be removed, the skin wrinkles, eyes need glasses. We take these signs of ageing for granted, never for one moment realizing that there are ways to correct certain forms of refractive error, especially those which occur in the young.

The experiences of many people disprove the notion that eye problems are inevitable and incurable and yoga is playing a large part in this revolution. Aldous Huxley, the famous author, was nearly blinded at the age of sixteen by *keratitis punctato*, a condition caused by opacities of the cornea and made worse by farsightedness and astigmatism. After a few months of special eye exercises he was able to read without glasses and without strain.

Dr William Bates was an ophthalmologist who lived in the early part of this century and who presented a revolutionary method of visual re-education. As a young doctor Bates did not believe that glasses were the only answer. Forty years of research resulted in a sophisticated technique that has proven effective in many cases. He developed the theory that defective vision is not inherited but occurs when mental and emotional stress cause the eyes to be strained. He devised a system of exercises and a relaxation technique similar to yoga nidra. Through his techniques, flashes of vision occur which increase in clarity and length over a period of time until clarity replaces fuzziness. To understand how this can occur we need to know a little more about the cause of eye defects.

The underlying cause

The lens is controlled by ciliary muscles which accommodate vision to far and near objects. Contraction of these muscles occurs when we look at near objects, causing the lens to thicken, increasing its power. When we look into the distance, the normal eye adjusts the ciliary muscles within a fraction of a second. This adjustment proceeds with incredible precision to give us a constantly clear image of the world.

In short-sightedness the ciliary muscles are constantly contracted, in spasm, preventing the lens from accommodating to distant objects. Spasm is caused by straining to see. For example, short-sightedness is very common in young students who are constantly straining while reading, thereby forcing the ciliary muscles to contract for abnormally long periods of time. It is not reading which is the problem, but the straining to read and understand, long hours, fatigue and an unhealthy, imbalanced lifestyle. Many students live in a world of near objects and their eyes 'forget' how to adjust to long distances. This may be one of the reasons myopia is so common in the young.

Straining to see or read, or in any other use of the eyes, is often accompanied by straining of the other facial muscles, forehead, temples, jaw muscles and also of the neck and shoulders. Myopia and other eye defects then fall into the category of general mental and emotional tensions and can be regarded as psychosomatic disorders.

Another interesting facet of facial tension and refractive errors is the fact that we forget to blink, and this intensifies straining. Blinking is vital for maintaining moist, healthy eyes and for protecting the eyes from foreign objects, such as dust and grit. At the same time blinking momentarily rests the eyes. When we strain, the blinking mechanism also suffers. It is an interesting exercise to sit and blink consciously a few times in order to experience its effect on the state of tension within the eyes.

By far the most common refractive error of the elderly is hypermetropia. As age creeps up, the ciliary muscles weaken and it becomes difficult for them to contract sufficiently to allow the lens to accommodate for near objects. It is also quite common for myopic eyes to become normal for some time before hypermetropia takes over. Many people find themselves in the situation where they are unable to focus on either far or near objects and require bi-focal lenses, the upper lens for distance and the lower for reading.

A medical examination is essential to exclude such conditions as diabetes, high blood pressure, arteriosclerosis or nephritis, which are also common causes of poor eyesight.

Correcting the error
The obvious means of correcting the tension and weakness of the refracting muscles of the eye is to institute a series of exercises to initially relax and then to strengthen, not

only the muscles themselves, but also our control over these muscles. At the same time we must work on our general body tensions. This is a much more sensible method of approaching the situation than glass lenses, which tend to splint the eye defect and prevent its returning to a normal state. If we become dependent on glasses we will never be able to see without them.

Along with exercises for the eyes, a health promoting lifestyle is necessary. Diet should be simple, light and free from chemicals and refined and processed foods. Certain vitamins are particularly important for good vision. These include vitamin A, found in yellow carotene containing food groups, such as carrots and apricots, vitamin B2 and the essential amino acid tryptophane, found in milk, and Vitamin C, found in fresh fruit and vegetables. These nutrients are particularly important for children.

Asana

The following exercises neutralize eyestrain and teach us the correct use of all eye muscles. They help smooth out the distortion of the lens and the eye itself, and should be incorporated into our daily routine.

The chapter in *Asana Pranayama Mudra Bandha*, published by Yoga Publications Trust, entitled 'Yoga Exercises for the Eyes' is a complete guide for eye health and for the eye conditions mentioned in this chapter, as well as for many other eye conditions. Some or all of the exercises can be performed at any time of day. For example, palming can be practised any time the eyes are tired or when you feel fatigued. The exercises act on the internal ciliary muscles as well as on the external muscles responsible for eye movement. Palming, front and sideways viewing, and distant and near viewing are all particularly good for the ciliary muscles.

Shambhavi mudra, which is incorporated into the above series, is by itself a powerful redirector of pranic and psychic energies. It stimulates ajna chakra, the third eye, and by stimulating this centre of higher intuitive awareness, it allows

13

us insight into the very potent factors at the mental and psychic levels which are causing refractive errors in the first place. It relaxes tension by stimulating the optic centre, a powerful generator of alpha brainwaves, which are associated with relaxation. By just crossing the eyes alpha waves are generated. Shambhavi mudra leads us into meditative states and awakens inner vision, awareness of the spiritual dimension.

Palming is also a relaxing, alpha producing exercise in which heat produced by rubbing the palms of the hands is used to soothe the eyes. At the same time we gaze into the infinite dark space of *chidakasha*, feeling that our eyes are melting and releasing all their tensions. The same relaxing effect can be obtained by sitting with the eyes closed while facing the rising or setting sun. The rays of the sun will be felt to penetrate deep into the eyes, associated with a very pleasant sensation. In both exercises avoid any concentration. Simply gaze and allow all tension to melt away.

While performing the palming exercise, it is useful to place a card one or two feet (30–60 cms) in front of the face with a number or some symbol inscribed on it. While palming, mentally visualize the symbol clearly, as though one were actually seeing it with great clarity and minus any fuzziness. After a few minutes remove the hands, open the eyes and gaze gently at the symbol which should appear quite clearly for a few seconds before the old muscular habits reassert themselves. This will retrain the muscles over time.

Sirshasana and sarvangasana are useful to promote circulation to the eyes. Surya namaskara and surya bheda pranayama remove physical tensions, stimulate pingala nadi, supply us with extra physical energy and so help promote healing of the whole physical body.

Hatha yoga shatkarma

Neti kriya acts directly on the olfactory and ocular systems, affecting all the structures of the face via reflex nervous activity. It is a particularly soothing and pleasant practice as well as being immensely practical. One medical practitioner has reported that it has proven useful even in the treatment of trachoma, an infection of the eyes which often leads to blindness. Neti is useful in all ocular conditions, as well as for headaches, neurological disorders and coughs and colds. It acts on ajna chakra and awakens prana in the facial area, thereby reducing tension in all the facial musculature as well as in the whole body-mind complex.

Amaroli benefits the eyes, especially when fresh midstream urine, which may be diluted according to individual needs, is dropped directly into the eyes. Urine neti (diluted with water) may also be performed. If amaroli practice proves difficult, fresh water may be substituted.

Trataka is a very powerful yogic shatkarma, which is especially useful in myopia. If your vision improves when you squint, or when you gaze through the tiny hole made by curling the first finger of the hand, then trataka on a black spot will be of immense benefit. Trataka is the best method of uprooting the habit of straining and staring, replacing it by gentle, controlled gazing. It acts on the whole optic system and steadies the turbulent and erratic flow of the neurotic, anxious mind. We know that in anxiety and mental tension, the eyes shift about and are unsteady. In some cases the individual cannot look directly into the eyes of the person to whom he or she is talking. Mental tensions are the root cause of many eye disorders, acting on the internal as well as external eye musculature. When the gaze is steadied, the mind as well as the muscles relax. The practice of trataka has a very powerful influence on many levels of our personality.

A modified or adapted form of trataka is called central fixation. The normal eye forms images around the central point of the retina, called the macula lutea or light spot. The rest of the field of vision is vague and less well defined. We can become aware of the process especially during reading or writing. While reading, aim to keep vision just below the line being read. As the eye shifts from one side to the other, be aware that the word nearest the point of central fixation appears more distinct than the others. While writing, be aware of the pen tip where clarity is greatest as well as the rest of the page. This tends to expand the field of vision, so that we can take in not only the central area but also the outer, less well-defined spaces. Relaxation occurs.

Relaxation
Yoga nidra is one of the most scientific methods of relaxation yet devised. It acts at the deepest levels of our being, reducing those tensions which cause most of our diseases and problems in life. In dealing with eye problems directly, we can spend more time working on the eyes and facial structures during the rotation of consciousness in the body. During breath awareness the movement of the breath should be felt in the facial region, or as coming in and out of ajna chakra and moving in a line from *bhrumadhya*, the eyebrow centre, to the back of the head. A triangle can also be visualized, with the nostrils and the eyebrow centre as the three corners. The breath can be felt flowing up the sides, from the nostrils to the eyebrow centre and back down again.

A combination of the above methods is a powerful approach to remove refractive errors, to regain normal vision and to awaken inner vision and higher intuitive awareness.

Headache

Headache is one of the most common symptoms a doctor is asked to treat. There are several types of headache, and the origin of pain is slightly different for each one. The brain itself is insensitive to pain, but many other structures both inside and outside of the skull have sensitive pain fibres. These include the arteries and venous sinuses of the brain, the dura mater or membrane surrounding the brain and the external scalp muscles.

Clinical features

There are some causes of headache which should be treated by a medical expert, such as tumours, meningitis or acute fevers. The types of headache described below also have a number of different causes. Therefore, in all cases of chronic headache a medical check up is essential.

- *Vascular headaches* are the typically throbbing type and are due to dilation of blood vessels. The headache which accompanies fever and systemic infections is typical. It is due to dilation of the intracranial blood vessels, as are throbbing headaches which occurs at high altitude or which follow a blow to the head, an epileptic fit or excessive consumption of alcohol.
- *Migraine and hypertension headaches*, on the other hand, are thought to be due to dilation of the extracranial arteries, outside the skull.

- *Muscle spasm* is one of the most common causes of headache. The muscles of the scalp or the neck go into a spasm due to emotional tension. This produces persistent and continuous type of headache which varies in intensity from a feeling of tightness to a true pain. It is usually bilateral. Painful, tender areas can often be felt in the tight scalp muscles, or in the neck muscles. Cervical spondylitis and poor spinal posture in general are frequent causes.
- *Referred headache* from the eyes is also common. It often accompanies eyestrain and glaucoma. Similarly, inflammation or irritation of the sinuses and nasal passages often manifest as a headache.
- *Psychogenic headache* is the term used to describe headcaused by emotional or mental tensions. It is often a vascular or tension headache, being experienced as a sense of pressure at the top of the head, or as a tight band around the scalp. Migraine belongs in this group.

The most common headaches

The two most common forms of headache are migraine and tension headaches.

Migraine: This severe form of headache occurs more commonly in women than men. It is characterized by periodic headaches which are usually one-sided and are often accompanied by visual disturbances and vomiting. Migraine is thought to be caused by swelling of the arteries outside the skull due to instability of the autonomic nervous system which controls the flow of blood into the head. Pain is caused by the stretching of pain nerve endings in the arterial wall.

Migraine is found to have a family predisposition, with three in four migraine sufferers having close relatives who are similarly affected. It is uncertain whether this predisposition is genetic or is behaviourally inherited.

Migraine usually starts after puberty and continues until late middle life. Acute attacks are often related to emotional stress, occasionally occurring during the period of relaxation when the stress appears to be over. Attacks occur at intervals varying from a few days to several months. The first symptom of an attack is commonly a sensation of white or coloured lights, moving spots, wavy lines or visual defects. Loss of sensation or weakness of one half of the body may be experienced or there may be numbness of both hands and around the mouth. These symptoms may last up to half an hour. This period is known as the 'migrainous aura'. It is followed by the actual pain of the headache, which usually begins in one spot and subsequently involves the whole of one or occasionally both sides of the head. The pain is usually severe and throbbing in character, and is associated with vomiting, photophobia (aversion to light), pallor, sweating and prostration, which may cause severe loss of muscle tone and necessitate the patient taking to bed in a darkened room. The attack may last from a few hours to several days, leaving the patient weak and exhausted.

A migraine attack may be precipitated by many factors, but for each sufferer there is usually a characteristic one. It may be a response to a particular food, especially the tyramine rich foods, such as cheese, chocolate and red wine. It is not always easy to locate the cause immediately but the sufferer should seek to locate factors which precipitate the attack.

Similarly, there are many phases of migraine. Some people have migraine with the rising sun, and it gets better as the sun falls towards the horizon. They may be completely free of attack when conditions are cloudy. In other people, the incidence of migraine appears to be related to the lunar cycle. The site of migraine attack also varies. Some sufferers will experience the attack in only half of the head, while other sufferers experience the pain at the top or at the back of the head.

Tension headaches: Tension headaches are related to migraine but manifest through the somatic nervous system instead of through the autonomic nervous system. These headaches are produced by sustained contractions of the external scalp muscles. These headaches are usually constant and non-pulsatile and may be unilateral or bilateral. The sufferer often describes a feeling like a tight band around the head, or a feeling of the head being in a vice or under great pressure. Migraines usually last for a few hours, but may extend much longer. With prolonged headache, the muscles of the head, jaws, neck and upper back may become tender and tight and movement may be limited. In addition, hardened, localized, painful areas in the scalp muscles commonly arise. Generally poor posture is a major factor.

Tension headaches commonly follow emotional stress, but sustained muscle contraction may also be a factor in the pain associated with vascular headaches, and with diseases of the eyes, ears, nose, teeth and sinuses. Similarly, the type of headache which is found to be associated with cervical arthritis (spondylitis) or disc degeneration generally stems from muscular spasm.

Tension headaches and migraine often occur in the same person. Headache is also a common symptom of constipation and menstrual irregularity. These headaches disappear when the underlying condition is recognized and treated.

Medical treatment of headaches

Many headaches disappear when an underlying cause such as fever, eye disorders, or sinusitis has been removed. Others may respond well to osteopathic treatment or removal of allergenic foods. Otherwise the treatment is symptomatic, as conventional medical science has been unable to provide a cure for psychogenic headaches such as migraine or tension headache.

Symptomatic treatment using various drugs which provide temporary relief is all that is currently prescribed in the first instance. Muscle tension headaches sometimes respond to aspirin or tranquillizers, psychotherapy, massage and heat. For migraine type vascular headaches the commonly prescribed drugs are derived from ergot alkaloids. These must be taken at the first sign of the attack if they are to be of any benefit. Rectal aspirin suppositories also help. In general, however, the medical management of chronic, persistent headache symptoms at the present time is fairly ineffective, and the conditions present a real problem for both the patient and the doctor.

Yogic management

Yogic practices fill the gap in managing these types of headache which medical science finds difficult to treat. Psychogenic headache, vascular headaches, including migraine, and muscle tension headache can often be eradicated completely through yogic practices alone.

Fundamental practices for migraine and tension headaches are the hatha yoga shatkarmas, kunjal and neti. If they are performed at the beginning of an attack of migraine, the sufferer gains immediate relief. These practices release the build-up of psycho-emotional tension which is precipitating the attack. In eradicating headaches these shatkarmas should be practised daily each morning, in conjunction with the following program for two or three months.

1. *Asana*: Pawanmuktasana part 1, surya namaskara.
2. *Pranayama*: Bhramari, nadi shodhana, gentle bhastrika.
3. *Shatkarma*: Kunjal and neti daily. Laghoo shankhaprakshalana once a week. Shankhaprakshalana (full practice) should be undertaken in an ashram environment preferably before commencing the program.
4. *Relaxation*: Yoga nidra daily.
5. *Diet*: A simple vegetarian diet is recommended. Avoid rich foods, especially cheese, chocolate and wine. Avoid over-eating.
6. *Fasting*: Skipping a meal and relaxing for ten minutes in shavasana will often avert an impending headache if it is due to mental stress.

Thyroid Disease

We all know people who can eat and eat and never get fat, while others need only to think of food to put on weight. Some people fly through the day with energy and vitality to spare while others have to drag their bodies around like dead weights. These are all examples of variations in metabolism, the energy system of the physical body.

Metabolism

Metabolism is the sum total of the conservation and expenditure of all body energies and is divided into two:

1. *Anabolism*: The build-up and replacement of tissues and the storage of energy; for example, glucose is taken from the digestive tract and stored in the liver as glycogen.
2. *Catabolism*: The breakdown of tissues and the use of energy.

The process of metabolism is extremely complex and science has not yet found the keys to unlock all its mysteries. It is known, however, that the thyroid gland is the regulator of metabolism in the body and is itself regulated by the pituitary gland in the skull. Regulation of metabolism in a healthy person occurs in response to physical and emotional demands relayed through the brain and its hypothalamic centres.

The thyroid

The thyroid gland lies in the front of the neck, wrapped around the trachea. It is divided into two lobes, one on either side of the neck, and secretes hormones into the blood-stream. These hormones, which are called thyroxin (T4) and triiodothyronine (T3), determine our metabolic rate. Their manufacture depends upon the presence of various nutrients, including essential fatty acids, the amino acid tyrosine, zinc and iodine. The absence of any of these substances can lead to underactive thyroid function and cause an enlargement of the thyroid gland, known as goitre. This occurs most commonly in mountainous areas, such as the Himalayas, and other regions far from the sea.

Thyroid diseases

In regions where there are no obvious deficiencies of the essential nutrients, thyroid disorders are still very common. Here, the two major forms of thyroid diseases are hyperthy-roidism (overactive thyroid) and hypothyroidism (under-active thyroid).

Hyperthyroid or thyrotoxicosis: In this condition the gland secretes excess hormones. It is eight times more likely to be found in women than in men, and most commonly between the ages of thirty and fifty. Thyrotoxic individuals become thin, tremulous, irritable, anxious and even hysterical. Because the metabolism is raised, they experience rapid heart rate and palpitations, rapid shallow respirations, frequent bowel motions and diarrhoea, flushing, heat intolerance, sweating, menstrual disturbance, and sometimes bulging of the eyes (exophthalmos). Such people suffer the paradoxical situation in which they feel fatigue and lack of energy and yet they are compulsively active. They are restless and fidgety and the slightest remark may set off an inap-propriately angry response.

Conventional medical management of this condition includes drugs, such as carbimazole, radioactive iodine and surgery.

Hypothyroidism: This condition occurs when there is insufficient hormone secretion. The symptoms of hypothy-roidism are those of decreased metabolism with the slowing of mental and physical activities, constipation, slowing of movement, tiredness, vague muscle pains, deafness, hoarseness, weight gain despite poor appetite, dry skin and hair, disordered menstruation and forgetfulness.

The onset of this disease is gradual and its symptoms are often mistaken for signs of ageing. Listlessness, dullness and apathy can be so marked that the patient does not care for herself or even want treatment, having to be persuaded by family or friends to seek medical assistance. Frequently the doctor will recognize the condition on meeting the patient by chance after a long interval. An advanced case characteristically has swollen, puffy eyelids, thick lips and an enlarged tongue. The skin retains fluid, becoming pale and turgid, sweating is absent and the skin is flabby and dry, the speech slow, monotonous and husky. Later in the disease, heart failure occurs. The replacement of thyroid hormone in these patients has dramatic effects.

Holistic medical management of thyroid disorders

Both underactive and overactive thyroid dysfunctions are autoimmune disorders. This means that our immune system is producing antibodies to our own tissues. There is increasing evidence that when our digestion is not functioning properly and the food is not broken down fully in the gut, the incompletely digested proteins become immunogenic; that is, they are large enough for the immune system to recognize them as foreign entities and produce antibodies for protection. Unfortunately, the antibodies can cross-react with our own tissues and in this case attack the thyroid gland.

A comprehensive assessment by a physician skilled in both allopathic and naturopathic therapy could be very beneficial.

Yogic management

The thyroid is also related to vishuddhi chakra, the psychic centre which purifies the poisons of the body, *vish*, and turns them into *amrit*, the nectar of immortality. Long before medical science ever knew about the existence of thyroid glands, the yogis had devised practices which not only maintained healthy glands and metabolism, but also formed part of a system of enlightenment. The good health of the neuroendocrine system was understood to be vital to higher awareness.

Sarvangasana (shoulder stand) is the most well recognized asana for the thyroid gland. An enormous pressure is placed on the gland by this powerful posture. As the thyroid has one of the largest blood supplies of any body organ, this pressure has dramatic effects on its function, improving circulation and squeezing out stagnant secretions. Stimulation of the area draws the awareness to the area, and with attentive awareness comes prana, the vehicle of healing. This means that as we concentrate on the area, the sensory nerves are stimulated, setting relays within the brain into motion. As the whole process is health giving, the brain tends to readjust its regulatory centres and a corresponding readjustment of muscular states, blood flow and nervous activity in the neck area follows. Therefore, the practice of sarvangasana is useful in both mild over and under-active states, as its overall effect is to rebalance. The effects of sarvangasana are enhanced by feeling the normal breath moving in and out of the throat while in this position.

After sarvangasana, we should perform matsyasana, and from sarvangasana we can practise halasana, pashinee mudra, padma sarvangasana, and other variations. All these practices are positive influences for better health of the thyroid gland. At the same time, all these practices should be avoided in severe thyrotoxicosis, physical debility or a very enlarged goitre, where medical therapy is obviously the first line of treatment to be given.

Vipareeta karani mudra, though not placing as much pressure on the thyroid gland area, is more powerful than sarvangasana because it incorporates ujjayi pranayama and awareness of psychic passages. It is also more useful in goitre, though once again adding iodine to the diet is the first obvious step.

25

Other effective asanas include surya namaskara, pawan-muktasana with emphasis on the head and neck exercises, yoga mudra, supta vajrasana and all backward bending asanas, sirshapada bhumi sparshasana, kandharasana, grivasana, simhagarjanasana. Pawanmuktasana is useful for initial therapy in severe thyroid disease and for older patients.

The most effective pranayama for thyroid problems is ujjayi. It acts on the throat area and its relaxing and stimulating effects are most probably due to stimulation of ancient reflex pathways within the throat area (associated, for example, with vomiting, breathing, swallowing) which are controlled by the brain stem and hypothalamus. This practice also gives us direct access into the pranic and psychic networks, the substructure of metabolic activity. Ujjayi is the basis of vishuddhi shuddhi and ajapa japa, which are very powerful yogic procedures and should be taught after the patient has acquired the initial skills thoroughly.

Nadi shodhana pranayama is useful in rebalancing metabolism through its effects on ida and pingala. Sheetali and seetkari, cooling breaths, are valuable in the hyperthyroid state in order to cool the overactive hypermetabolic and therefore overheated body. Bhastrika pranayama should be used in hypothyroidism because of its heating effects, its ability to speed up metabolism.

Jalandhara bandha applies pressure to the thyroid area and should be incorporated into pranayama cautiously and after the initial exercises have been mastered. Other bandhas can also be added to enhance the effects of pranayama. Of course, in the long run the most powerful techniques to tune not only the thyroid gland, but also the whole neuroendocrine system, are the potent maha bandha, maha mudra, and maha bheda mudra. These can be mastered only by advanced yoga students.

The role of emotional relaxation

One of the most prominent precipitating factors in states of thyroid imbalance is long-term suppression and blockage of emotional expression. This is closely related to another

26

condition, 'globus hystericus', which is also prominent in middle-aged women. Here the major symptom is the frequent desire to swallow so as to remove a psychic lump or tensions in the throat area. In yogic treatment this constant, sustained tension is sometimes experienced consciously for the first time during the deeper stages of yoga nidra, as the three-fold accumulated and deeply set tensions – muscular, mental and emotional – are progressively ended up.

Balancing of the emotions, and giving a suitable outlet for their expression is an important part of yoga therapy for thyroid disease. Kirtan (singing of mantras collectively to the point of self-forgetfulness and transcendence) is one of the most useful means. Another is ajapa japa meditation (practice of mantra awareness in the frontal psychic passage from navel to throat) in conjunction with ujjayi pranayama.

Cardiovascular System

The Heart and Circulatory System

Cardiac (heart) disease and arteriosclerosis (blood vessel degeneration) are the largest killers in the affluent sectors of world society today. Every year, many millions of people die from the complications of cardiovascular degeneration – including hypertension, chronic heart failure, stroke (cerebro-vascular accident), and kidney disease. In addition, many more experience the anguish of chest pains known as angina pectoris, which indicate cardiac strain in the activities of their daily life.

The causes and effects of heart strain are many and complex, involving the nervous system, through which mental and emotional processes influence the cardiac function, and the metabolic, digestive and reproductive systems, which frequently place excessively heavy demands upon the heart.

The heart and circulatory system or the heart of the matter

The heart is a unique neuromuscular pump which is at the centre of all human activity. It is responsible for maintaining the circulation of blood throughout the body. Every part of the body is dependent upon the heart, and if it ceases to work, the whole body ceases to function within a few minutes. The heart beats untiringly, night and day, from the beginning of life to the last, dying breath. When the body rests, it beats quietly and slowly. When exercising, the heart immediately quickens its pace to increase the volume of blood reaching the distant muscles and cells.

The power of the heart depends on the fibres in its muscular walls. Damage to these fibres produces striking changes in the pattern and efficiency of blood circulation. Many factors are responsible for maintaining the volume and pressure of the blood. These include the condition of the heart valves, the influence of the nervous system in controlling the internal diameter of the blood vessels, and the amount of fluid in the bloodstream. However, the primary condition of the heart muscle is most important of all.

The heart is composed of a unique type of muscle known as cardiac muscle, which is more durable than any other muscular tissue in the body. It enables the heart to continue its repetitive function ceaselessly, without faltering. No other organ works as long or as hard as the heart.

The arterial circulation

The blood circulates from the heart to the body through a complex network of conducting pipeways known as arteries, veins and capillaries. Arteries are the largest and strongest type of blood vessels. They distribute freshly oxygenated blood from the heart to the smaller blood vessels, called capillaries. They may become hardened so that the elastic tissue in their walls loses its flexibility. This can constrict the arteries, raise the blood pressure and thereby increase the work of the heart. It may also lead to insufficient oxygen supply to the heart itself and to other body organs.

The chambers of the heart

The inside of the heart is composed of four chambers. Blood containing a rich supply of oxygen arrives from the lungs to be distributed to the body. It first enters the left atrium or upper chamber, and flows from this chamber into the larger left ventricle. This is the chamber upon which most of the blood circulation depends. The instant the left ventricle begins to contract, the mitral valve snaps shut, closing the connecting door to the left atrium. At almost the same instant, the aortic valve opens, allowing blood to rush through the aorta to the other arterial branches of the body.

The coronary arteries

All main arteries of the body branch off from the aorta. The first two branches are known as the coronary arteries, which are about five inches (12 cms) long and 1/8 inch (3 mm) in diameter. These arteries are responsible for supplying blood to the left and right sides of the heart muscles itself. If one of them should become narrowed, the whole of the circulation system may fail, as the muscle fibres of the heart itself are deprived of nourishing oxygen. In a healthy person there is always sufficient blood flowing into these arteries to meet the needs of the heart, but sometimes they become partially or totally blocked. This can be caused by blood clots, constriction due to nervous spasm or hardening of the vessel walls. In these cases, heart attack and heart failure can occur. Degeneration of the blood vessel walls is termed arteriosclerosis. It is related to an animal fat diet, cigarette smoking, lack of exercise and excessive mental stress and strain.

Regular practice of yoga can relieve and prevent this disease by eliminating unnecessary tension from our lives. Sensible dietary habits are also necessary as part of a yogic lifestyle.

The venous return

The right atrium and right ventricle operate in a similar way to the left atrium and left ventricle. They pump oxygen-depleted blood, filled with carbon dioxide wastes, to the lungs. This blood, that has deposited its oxygen in the cells of the body, flows back to the right side of the heart through the network of veins, and is pumped into the lungs. In the lungs it gives up the carbon dioxide wastes from the distant cells and these are expelled from the body with expiration. In exchange, a fresh supply of oxygen is taken up, and this blood flows back to the left side of the heart to be pumped out to the cells of the body once again.

The work capacity of the heart

The amount of work done by the heart in one day is almost beyond belief. For life to continue, the process of circulation must go on ceaselessly. The heart must pump, 24 hours a day, 50–80 times a minute, from birth to death. When the heartbeat stops, life automatically ceases. This amounts to 100,000 contractions in one day, or 37 million times in one year. In an average lifespan of seventy years, this amounts to two and a half billion beats. No man-made machine has such reliability and durability.

Like any other pump, the heart is subject to wear and tear, especially if it is abused and overstrained. The key to a long life lies in preserving the heart from excessive strain of all kinds. This must include preservation of mental and emotional balance, dietary control, adequate exercise and sleep, and is best attained by following a yogic lifestyle.

If the heart has been damaged by disease, it will repair itself while it works. If its valves become thickened because of disease, such as rheumatic fever, the muscular walls of the heart will thicken in an attempt to compensate for any loss of efficiency. Under the stress of extreme exercise or fever, it will go on pumping at a rate of up to two to three times its normal speed to enable the body to overcome the crisis.

The pacemaker

The rate at which the heart beats is governed by the pacemaker or SA node, a small fragment of specialized nervous tissue located near the top right side of the heart. This node generates a spontaneous rhythmic electrical impulse which is conducted throughout the upper chambers of the heart and then on to all the muscle fibres, initiating the cardiac contraction. Thus the heartbeat is controlled by the output of impulses from the pacemaker, which is in turn governed by the ever changing needs of the body.

The seat of human emotion

The heart's function is intimately related to our emotional metabolism. Our emotional states directly influence the behaviour of the heart, and heart disease is often as much an emotional disorder as a physical disease. An anxious, overtense mind, always gripped by worries and problems or an unruly mind, constantly bursting into habitual states of anger, passion or sorrow, causes wild, uncontrolled activation of the sympathetic nervous system and floods the circulation with the stress hormones, adrenalin and noradrenalin. The heart rate is elevated above its optimal resting state, which subjects it to strain.

Similarly, the stresses of interpersonal relationships, encompassing the expression of the whole range of human emotions, instincts and desires which must be experienced as we evolve, place constant demands upon the heart and the endocrine glands. When the expression of the passions and unruly emotions is uncontrolled and unmanageable, hormonal secretions become imbalanced and wayward, and the heart labours excessively. Sympathetic activation is also responsible for sending the small arteries into a state of spasm or permanent contraction. Consequently, the heart must pump against a high back pressure of blood in the arterial tree, and hypertension (high blood pressure) inevitably results.

Hypertension is a serious and damaging disorder, accelerating blood vessel damage, leading to kidney and heart failure, and posing the constant threat of sudden death by stroke (bursting of a blood vessel in the brain).

Until recently doctors believed that heart attack (myocardial infarction) was caused by a blood clot lodging in one of the coronary arteries. However, it is now accepted that in many cases of heart attack, there is probably no blood clot, and that the attack is a functional crisis in the nervous system, caused by a spasm of the coronary arteries, and is due to overactivation of the sympathetic nervous system. The same applies to angina, a chronic, ongoing form of partial ary occlusion where spasm of the coronary arteries is an important factor.

It now appears that in both these common heart diseases, the most important precipitating cause is spasm of the coronary artery, caused by high levels of mental tension acting through the automatic nerve fibres that supply the arteries themselves.

Emotional tension is one prominent cause of heart attack. Most coronary patients are found to have suffered a deep and significant emotional hurt or disappointment during the month before, or even one year before, the heart attack.

Relation of cardiac and sexual functions

Both our emotions and our instincts demand an outlet, and this commonly occurs via the sexual behaviour. The human reproductive system is controlled by the pituitary (master control) gland.

The pituitary gland is controlled by the hypothalamus releasing hormones from the brain which are synthesized in response to our various mental and emotional states. This means that the formation of semen in the male and the menstrual cycle in the female result directly from the emotional metabolism.

When certain types of emotions are elevated or are uncontrolled, high levels of the sexual hormones: testosterone in the male, and oestrogen and progesterone in the female, are synthesized by the gonads (testes and ovaries) and secreted into the bloodstream. These hormones activate the reproductive and sexual organs, which become the mediums for emotional expression and release.

Men are far more likely to suffer from vascular and degenerative heart disease than women, up to the age of menopause. Researchers believe that it is high levels of the androgenic or masculine hormones which are responsible both for the characteristic aggressiveness of the 'cardiac personality', and for damage to the vessels of the heart itself in coronary disease.

in his field and has done well in life by driving himself to the limit. He sets high personal standards and expects others to conform to these same standards. He often becomes a 'workaholic', using his work as his sole means of self-fulfilment, while tending to avoid painful emotional encounters and responsibilities in the family.

While appearing a most strong-willed and independent character on the surface, his inner, subjective nature may be quite the opposite. He is frequently a highly sensitive, perceptive and even artistic person, but has suppressed this softer side of his personality. This contrast often leads to an inner conflict which lies at the root of heart strain and cardiac diseases.

In yogic therapy, it is often difficult for the cardiac personality to relax and utilize yoga in a non-competitive way. His mind is so achievement-orientated that relaxation and the attitude of letting go, surrender and acceptance is very unnatural for him at first. Nevertheless, if this lesson can be learned, progress is assured.

Yoga balances the emotions

Because the emotions play such a fundamental role in the genesis of cardiac diseases, it is not sufficient that a heart patient adopt a low fat diet alone in order to manage his condition.According to yogic science, it is essential for sufferers of cardiac strain or those recovering from cardiac crisis, to recognize their patterns of emotional response and the effects these have upon the heart and mind. This is achieved through the practices of yogic relaxation, yoga nidra and meditation (dhyana). Mastery of a scientific technique of relaxation like yoga nidra is the most important first step in recovery from cardiac crisis through yoga.

This is because heart patients are often very much ruled by their emotional states, even though they may appear on the surface to be very calm, cool and collected personalities. Suppressed emotions, which are held deep inside and denied expression for many years due to feelings of shame, guilt or rejection, are nevertheless registered as a continuing, excessive heart strain and are found to be major contributing factors in many heart diseases.

By practising yoga, the individual is gradually liberated from these deep emotional complexes, fears, and inadequacies which are harboured in the subconscious mind. Often they are the impressions of unpleasant experiences from early childhood. These may never enter conscious awareness, but they nevertheless generate a high level of floating anxiety in daily life, colouring interactions, responses, attitudes and decisions. This is a root cause of constant tension and also of constant strain upon the heart.

The yogic practices unburden the heart, leading one to regain a child's emotions and outlook on life: open, simple and spontaneous. This provides enormous mental and cardiac relief for the heart patient, who is frequently deeply entwined in the emotional complexes of fear, self-pity, aggression, betrayal or anger. As relaxation occurs, pent-up emotions are liberated and the patient gradually learns to live, think and feel simply and honestly and to express feelings openly. Personality disturbance, due to suppression, is avoided, and outbursts of anger, excitement or passion no longer overwhelm the mind and overtax the heart.

Imagine the deep relaxation the heart would experience if it were freed from lurking anxieties and subconscious tensions. That is what the cardiac patient needs more than anything else and that is what yogic meditation, relaxation and other practices bring about.

Inadequacy of medical solutions

Medical sciences have developed many powerful drugs to control the symptoms and effects of cardiac strain, hypertension and heart failure. These drugs are often life-saving in the acute situation of a heart attack or hypertensive crisis. They lower a dangerously high blood pressure, stabilize a rapidly failing heart or relieve the pain of excessive cardiac effort (angina). However, they can never be the total solution to the problem because they do not get to the fundamental cause of heart disease and correct it.

Many patients depend on drugs for relief of symptoms for years or even decades, without realizing or coming to terms with the root cause of their condition. They grow tired and die before understanding what is fundamentally wrong with their mental and cardiac health, living out the remainder of their lives in an atmosphere of increasing suffering and discomfort.

When the emotions are known, experienced and expressed consciously, with an increasing faculty of awareness, cardiac strain can be reduced at its origins. This is why it is essential for cardiac patients to practise yoga under careful guidance, in conjunction with their medical therapy. Then they can gradually recognize and evolve beyond the limitation which is causing their heart and circulatory system to degenerate and their mind to suffer.

Yoga offers the solution

Yoga offers a tried and proven method for alleviating the emotional conflicts which impose enormous strain upon the human heart and leads to heart disease and its complications. Yoga provides a way of life by which the heart can be maintained in optimal condition right up to the end of life, as well as a way of relieving cardiac strain and illness.

In order to relieve the heart of its continuing burden, the emotional conflicts, dependencies, needs must first be known, accepted, and expressed. Then, ultimately, they can be transcended. The emotional metabolism cannot simply be suppressed out of existence, because suppression leads to mental disorders and physical disease. However, by following the path of yoga systematically, the emotions can be known and expressed in a healthy, fulfilling way which is not detrimental to health and which preserves the heart from crisis.

Meditation is fundamental to yogic life. It gradually instils peace, stability and increasing awareness into the life of the individual who is trapped in the throes of pain, fear, insecurity and emotional agony which accompany heart disease. Meditation induces a change in both body and mind. The body temperature, metabolic rate and endocrine secretion patterns undergo a profound, spontaneous change, the mind becomes deeply relaxed, and the heart becomes very, very quiet. The emotions are not extinguished, but their expression alters. Gradually, the heart rejoices as if relieved of a tremendous burden and soars skyward, expressing emotion in a joyful, transcendental way, no longer limited by the instinctive personality.

Yogic program for heart and circulatory disease

A tired and overworked heart needs rest more than anything else, for rest enables the levels of vital energy, prana, to build up and begin the work of regeneration. Adequate rest should be coupled with asana and pranayama, a short walk each day and moderate lifestyle.

Asanas are vitally important, but should never be practised beyond capacity. The heart must never be strained, and at the slightest sign of distress or pain the practice of relaxation should supervene.

1. *Asana*: Begin with pawanmuktasana parts 1 and 2. These should be practised each morning, after a bath which should be cold in summer but warm in winter. If pawanmuktasana part 2 proves too hard, it should be omitted. Shavasana should be practised whenever tiredness supervenes, and there should never be any hurry to finish the practices. Yoga should be a source of rest, relief and relaxation which will gradually spill over and transform the whole life. These asanas should continue daily for at least two months. Then shakti bandha asanas, if possible, can be introduced, and the following major asanas are recommended: vajrasana, shashankasana (relaxing for several minutes), sarpasana, yoga mudra, bhu namanasana.

2. *Pranayama*: Pranayama is very important both in the initial recovery of a heart patient and in the subsequent

42

rehabilitation and rejuvenation period. Pranayama should never impose a strain on the heart and lungs. If it does, then its purpose has been defeated. It should be soothing to the anxious mind, relaxing to the excited nerves and stabilizing to the irregular heart and circulation. The most important practices are nadi shodhana techniques one and two, and ujjayi pranayama. Breath should be only slightly deeper than normal, without retention, either internal or external. It should be as natural and as quiet as possible, and the awareness should follow the inflowing and outflowing breath very closely. Watching the breath is watching the mind and great relief of tension and anxiety will be experienced immediately. Cardiac function improves and mental stability develops week by week. The heart benefits greatly from the more efficient oxygenation process and damaged tissues are rapidly repaired. Ten rounds of nadi shodhana and ten rounds of ujjayi pranayama are recommended.

3. *Yoga nidra*: Relaxation should be practised at regular intervals during the asana program. Shavasana, matsya kridasana or advasana can be adopted. The full practice of yoga nidra should be followed once a day.

4. *Meditation*: Meditation should be learned not as a discipline but as an enjoyable pastime for the cardiac patient. Especially while confined to bed in the initial phase of recovery, and later on during rehabilitation, it is most useful as a means of becoming aware of the physical, mental and emotional tensions which have wrought such havoc upon the cardiovascular system. The most suitable practices are ajapa japa using the mantra So-ham, and antar mouna (inner silence). These practices bring detachment from the mental processes, fears and imaginations which are the root cause of mental agitations and tensions.

5. *Shatkarma*: Jala neti is an excellent practice for the heart patient. It can be learned and practised even while still

confined to bed, and should be adopted every morning. Kunjal and laghoo shankhaprakshalana should not be adopted by the heart patient, at least for many months, as they impose a strain on the heart.

6. *Karma yoga*: Selfless service, where one works with all attention, care and creativity, but without regard to the returns, rewards or profits of this work, can be successfully adopted during recovery from a cardiac illness.

7. *Changing the lifestyle*: Heart attack and cardiac strain occur most frequently in people who have a very rajasic, active, competitive temperament. Businessmen who become obsessively involved in their work are prime candidates for heart attack, for they neglect to take time off for relaxation and cell rejuvenation. They neglect to include relaxing pastimes in their lifestyle, becoming totally dedicated to their job.

Many people have lost the ability to really relax and have replaced it with a concept of relaxation which is usually comprised of stimulating habits such as smoking, drinking and social activities which excite and exhaust rather than relax the cardiovascular system. Skipping sleep and overeating further tire out the heart, circulatory and nervous systems.

It is an important part of recuperation that the patient be isolated completely from work worries and stays, if possible, in an environment which is natural and restful. An ashram environment could be ideal. This is often the first total holiday such people have allowed themselves in many, many years. There they can be introduced to some new interests which are creative, relaxing and non-competitive, more in tune with natural cycles and processes. For example, simple manual work such as carpentry is often a revelation and a great joy to a person who has previously used his hands only to sign cheques! Similarly, simple gardening, where the rate of return on investment depends not on economic conditions but on the blessing and abundance of the earth, can often help an anxious, ambitious person to relax and accept a pace of life more in harmony with nature.

8. *Swadhyaya*: Study of various scriptures and inspiring lives of saints who have devoted themselves to the realization and service of the highest truth, rather than to the acquisition of material and emotional possessions, is often a revelation to the heart patient, setting an example for a whole new dimension of stress-free living.

9. *Bhakti yoga*: The channelling of emotional energy away from personal objectives, desires and attachments towards the universal Self or God can also bring relief to the cardiac patient. Chanting, kirtan and other kinds of singing can also be very relaxing for people whose emotions are often deeply entangled in a mesh of attachments. Release of personal emotional entanglement often provides immense relief and paves the way for full recovery.

10. *Diet*: Diet should be light, avoiding meat, excessive protein, milk and dairy products, oil and excessive spices. These should be replaced by whole grains, fruits and fresh vegetables. This will reduce obesity which imposes constant, excessive strain on the heart. Meal times should be regular and the avoidance of eating between meals should become a rule of life. Overeating must be avoided, as it undoubtedly strains the heart. The evening meal should be taken before 7 p.m. These rules ensure that the digestive organs are not continually overtaxed, and liberate energy from digestion into healing.

It is important that the heart patient avoid constipation, as this leads to pranic blockage in the digestive tract. Excessive straining at stool is also stressful for the heart and for this reason, only a light, semi-liquid diet is recommended following a cardiac crisis. Diet can be gradually normalized as cardiac function is restored, but oils and fats and dairy products should be resumed cautiously. Smoking should be discontinued.

The Respiratory System

Disorders of the
Respiratory System

The respiratory system consists of the nose, pharynx, epiglottis, trachea, bronchi and lungs; also the ribcage that protects the lungs, the diaphragm and intercostal muscles which pump air in and out of the chest, and the nervous connections to the brain which activate and control these muscles.

For descriptive purposes, the respiratory system is divided into the upper and lower respiratory tracts. The arbitrary dividing line between the upper and lower tracts is considered to be in the larynx or upper windpipe, at the level of the Adam's apple (thyroid cartilage) at the front of the neck.

However, this division should not be allowed to obscure the intimate relationship between diseases of the upper respiratory tract and diseases of the bronchi and lungs in the chest. For example, an upper respiratory infection such as the common cold or sinusitis may, under certain conditions, give rise to bronchitis, or even pneumonia in the lungs themselves.

The upper respiratory tract
The upper respiratory tract includes the nose, the nasal passages and sinuses (nasopharynx), and the voice-box (larynx). The nasal sinuses are hollow cavities which communicate with the nasal passages through narrow

49

openings. These openings are frequently blocked in nasal infection such as colds and sinusitis. Adequate drainage of infected sinuses is often prevented by inflammatory swelling of their mucous membranes, so healing is often slow and incomplete.

As air is inhaled, it passes through the nostrils, the larynx and into the trachea (windpipe). The air we breathe must be changed before it enters the lungs because it is generally too dry and often too cold. Such air would quickly dry out the lung tissue. Furthermore, in the surrounding air there are many pollutants such as smoke and dust, as well as millions of germs. Many of these impurities must be removed before the air enters the lungs, otherwise we would be easily susceptible to lung infection or the lungs would become hopelessly blocked with dust and dirt.

To counter these dangers, the body is provided with an air purifying and conditioning system. This begins in the nose, where hairs at the entrance to the nostrils screen out large particles of dust and debris. Deeper passages of the nose moisten and warm the descending air. Special bone structures are lined with a thick, spongy mucous membrane through which circulates a rich supply of blood. As air passes over these tissues it is warmed, like air passing over a radiator. On cold days the blood vessels dilate to produce more heat and on warm days they shrink.

Disorders of the upper respiratory tract include the common cold (acute coryza), sinusitis, hay fever, tonsillitis and swollen adenoids.

The mucous secreting mechanism

Although the inhaled air has been filtered, it still contains a potentially lethal burden of fine dust particles. To help remove them, the airways are lined with glands which secrete a sticky film of mucus that traps the dust particles. This dust-filled mucus would clog the air passages if it wasn't for their remarkable self cleaning system. Microscopic hairs, called cilia, propel the mucus and debris upward by their sweeping motion towards the throat or larynx, where it is either swallowed, being harmless in the digestive tract, or coughed into the mouth to be spat out.

The cough reflex

At times we tax the capacity of our cleaning mechanisms, for example, when the inhaled air contains irritating substances such as automobile or industrial fumes or when we smoke too much. In a futile effort to trap countless millions of smoke particles, the throat secretes excess mucus. The mucus itself becomes an irritant and must be coughed up. In a cough, air is trapped in the lungs by the glottis, the valve at the upper end of the trachea, which carries air to the lungs. When the valve opens suddenly, air rushes out with explosive force. Thus the cough, which we may consider a nuisance, is actually essential to life. It is an emergency cleaning measure which rids the body of toxic products.

The larynx prevents large inhaled particles from reaching the lower respiratory tract by means of the cough reflex, in addition to being the organ of voice production. It is a frequent site of infection and inflammation (laryngitis), resulting in symptoms of dry cough, hoarseness and sore throat.

The lower respiratory tract

The lower respiratory tract consists of the trachea, the bronchi and the lungs. The trachea or windpipe begins at the voice box and ends by dividing into two tubes, the right and left bronchi. Each bronchus, measuring about four inches (10 cms) in length, passes to a lung where it divides into successively smaller branches known as bronchioles. This branching network of respiratory passages is known as the 'the bronchial tree'. Its smallest branches communicate with a cluster of minute air sacs called alveoli. The broncho-pulmonary lobules so constituted form the basic structure of the lungs. These innumerable tiny air cells render the lung tissues spongy and elastic.

The alveoli look like the cells of a sponge or a honeycomb. Each alveolus has a cobweb-like covering of capillaries, so tiny that red blood cells must pass through them in single file. Through their gossamer walls the blood gives up waste carbon dioxide and takes on refreshing oxygen. The oxygen is then distributed to all parts of the body via the heart, and the carbon dioxide is simultaneously expelled from the lungs and body during exhalation. Every few minutes the body's entire supply of blood must pass through the pulmonary capillaries, and in the process its colour changes from dark blue to bright red. Day and night this all important work proceeds without interruption, providing the energy which sustains all of the life processes in the body.

Disorders of the lower respiratory tract include such diseases as bronchitis, asthma, croup, whooping cough, pneumonia, emphysema, lung cancer, tuberculosis, pleural effusion, pleurisy and pneumothorax.

The breathing process

Normally we breathe about fifteen times per minute, inhaling about half a litre of air each time. During exercise, when cells are hungry for oxygen, the rate and depth of respiration increases and the lungs take in ten or more times the oxygen supplied during rest.

Breathing itself is an intricate process. The lungs hang loosely in the chest, each in a separate compartment with the heart in between. Around the lungs is a partial vacuum. Therefore, when the chest is enlarged by muscular contraction, the vacuum tugs the lungs outward, thus sucking in air. Inhalation is performed by either or both of two methods: i) the abdominal wall expands outwards due to the descent of the diaphragm into the abdomen, or ii) the ribs expand upwards and outwards. The process of expiration is simply a recoil mechanism.

Thus inhalation is an active process, while exhalation is normally a passive one. However, in states of bronchial spasm and mucus plugging of the airways, such as occurs in asthma, air has to be actively expelled from the lungs in order to overcome the increased resistance of the airways.

Behind many instances of respiratory disorder are two bad habits. The first is breathing through the mouth rather than the nose, and the second is breathing in short, shallow pants without fully expanding the abdomen or chest. These habits of poor respiration give rise to many mental deficiencies and physical disorders. The yogic science of pranayama (control and manipulation of life energy) is a fundamental part of yogic therapy. It commences with full instruction in the art and science of breathing consciously and efficiently. The breath becomes the vehicle for energizing the body and mind and at the same time it is the doorway into the higher spiritual states of expanded awareness.

The yogic alternative

Yogic and medical science understand the respiratory system very differently. For example, yoga recognizes mucus discharge as a beneficial elimination of toxic wastes from the body and effectively promotes the cleansing process by using the hatha yoga shatkarmas in conjunction with heat promotion procedures. Because the symptoms of excessive mucus discharge usually arise in cold weather and at the change of season, the problem is recognized as one of imbalance of body heat.

The yogic approach to rectifying imbalance in the respiratory system is gradual and gentle, with the emphasis on redirecting subtle energies rather than on just gross physical manipulation. Unlike the surgical process of antral washout, in yogic science cleansing of the sinuses is accomplished readily and painlessly by jala neti kriya. In this practice, warm saline water is introduced into one nostril while the head is tilted, allowing all the sinuses to be cleared and washed out before the stream of water emerges from the other nostril. Cases of long standing sinusitis, for example, respond rapidly to neti kriya, which is fundamental to the

53

health of the upper respiratory tract. It should be performed twice a day, and more often if necessary to promote mucus elimination, by anyone who suffers from bouts of hay fever, allergy, middle ear infections, colds, eosinophilia, wheezy bronchitis or asthma.

The introduction of neti into medical practice will revolutionize current management of ear, nose and throat disorders, and the introduction of yoga into medical practice will open new doorways of approach to treating many respiratory diseases.

The Common Cold

The common cold or acute coryza, also termed catarrh, is quite a mild disorder of short duration. In its more severe form it is called influenza or 'flu'. It is a highly contagious condition and attacks produce only temporary immunity, especially when the general level of the body's resistance is low. Coryza frequently occurs after exposure to sudden cold conditions, drenching in rainwater, or change of season, especially during early spring, early winter and monsoon, where the body's internal thermostat is adjusting to the sudden environmental changes. We must remember that it is the natural tendency of a healthy body to periodically discharge surplus toxins, and a cold is one of the most usual forms of cleansing and readjustment. Symptoms such as cough, sneezing, nasal discharge, fever and sweating are all signs of elimination.

Other factors which can precipitate a cold are unsuitable diet, sluggish digestion, sedentary lifestyle, lack of exercise, reduced muscle tone and sluggish circulation.

Clinical features

The onset of a cold is usually sudden with a tickling sensation in the nose and back of the throat, accompanied by sneezing. The throat often feels dry and sore, and a cough is often present. The head feels 'stuffed–up', the eyes smart and there is a profuse, watery, nasal discharge, A chilling sensation is usually experienced in the beginning, followed by slight fever. The skin may become hot and dry and the sufferer feels thirst, dryness of the tongue and loss of appetite. The urine may be darkened and of decreased volume, and the bowels may become temporarily constipated.

In more severe cases there may be shifting pains in the back and limbs. The mucous membrane of the nose becomes swollen and the sufferer is then forced to breathe through the mouth. A thin, irritating secretion flows from the nose, making the edges of the nostrils tender and sore, due to the need for constant cleaning of the nose. The tear ducts and glands become swollen causing the eyes to weep and the conjunctivae to become inflamed and reddened. Both the senses of smell and taste are commonly lost and, if the pharynx is involved, the voice becomes husky and a sore throat develops. Often the inflammation extends to the eustachian tubes, which causes the hearing to be temporarily impaired as well.

Usually, within a day or two, the nasal secretion becomes more profuse and the swelling of the nasal mucosa subsides, affording some relief. The sufferer is able to breathe through the nostrils again and within four or five days the symptoms disappear. However, in more severe cases, there is bronchial irritation and cough as the inflammation makes its way down the bronchial tree into the lower respiratory tract.

Complication of acute coryza

There are rarely any bad effects from a simple bout of cold, provided proper preventive and therapeutic measures are adopted, but where resistance is low or general health is poor, complications may occur as the infection spreads to other parts of the body. Severe influenza epidemics have been known to be lethal, especially in young children and the elderly. The most common complications of a cold are:

1. *Secondary bacterial infection*, where the secretions become thick and purulent.
2. *Sinusitis*, infection in the sinuses which leads to swelling, congestion, obstruction and thick purulent (yellow) discharge.
3. *Middle ear infection*, (otitis media), causing fever, deafness

and ear pain, as bacterial infection spreads from the nasopharynx up the eustachian tubes.

4. *Lower respiratory infection*, may lead to tracheitis (inflammation of trachea), laryngitis (larynx), bronchitis (bronchi) and lobular pneumonia, as secondary bacterial infection descends down the bronchial tree into the lungs.

Yogic management of acute coryza

Medical science has not devised a cure for the common cold or flu and so relies on symptomatic relief, with the appropriate antibiotics to prevent complicating secondary bacterial infection. However, a cold is a disorder which can definitely be averted by natural means when the pranic energy or vital resistance of the body is high and the physiological functions are in balance.

Overeating (especially of the wrong foods) often precipitates or worsens a cold. A short fast, on the other hand, is often sufficient to avert an imminent cold. At the first sign of a cold or sore throat, which represents a slight pranic imbalance, one should miss a meal, practise neti and kunjal kriya, and some energizing pranayama. Then take a cup of hot tea with heating spices (ginger, pepper, cinnamon) and rest quietly, perhaps performing mouna (silence) to minimize the wastage of energy which is caused by talking. Almost certainly the cold will never eventuate. One should also remember that a cold is very contagious during the early stages, especially when sneezing is prominent. Voluntary isolation and rest by the sufferer during this period is an important step.

If, however, the usual heavy meal is taken and work continues, prana will be further depleted. By proceeding with normal activities without any consideration for the impending cold, beyond maybe taking aspirin, one will almost certainly succumb by the next day to a full-blown cold, which may continue unabated for five days or more.

Many cases of cold are so mild, however, the sufferer continues on with the daily routine as usual. In this case, kunjal daily and neti once, twice or even thrice daily should remove stuffiness, cough and discomfort. Asana and pranayama should be minimized but meditation can be continued. However, if fever and constitutional disturbances occur, one should immediately retire to bed, taking six or more glasses of hot water with lemon juice during the day. Kunjal and neti should not be performed if a fever is present. The patient's yoga sadhana should definitely be confined to yoga nidra practice and antar mouna only.

Problems of recurrent common cold

People who experience colds or coryza several times a year, almost certainly have an impairment of their immune system. This can be due to any number of factors, including food allergies, vitamin and/or mineral deficiencies and, very commonly, protein deficiency which, in itself, may be due to inadequate dietary intake or an inability to digest, absorb or metabolize the food.

Yoga practices, which improve the digestive fire, the breathing pattern and overall immunity, as well as advice from a competent healthcare professional, will inevitably resolve this problem.

Further recommendations

- A light natural diet with plenty of fruit is advised, and for weakened patients, a liquid diet is best. Hot soup prepared from seasonal vegetables, such as carrot, spinach and tomato, can be made, together with coriander leaves, chilli and ginger. Foods rich in vitamins C and A are useful.
- Steam inhalation for ten minutes is advised in cases of nasal congestion and obstruction. This cleans the head and eases the breathing. In cases of cough, and sore and inflamed throat, gargling with warm saline water is useful.
- Smoking is irritative to the nasal mucosa and should be discontinued.
- Regular practice of surya namaskara to capacity builds up resistance to coughs and colds.

Bronchitis and Eosinophilia

Bronchitis is infection and inflammation of the mucous lining of the trachea and bronchi. It exists in both acute and chronic forms and usually develops as a sequel to upper respiratory infections such as cold or influenza. Other factors predisposing to bronchitis include cold, damp living conditions, foggy and dusty atmospheres, smoking and chronic mouth breathing, which allow unfiltered and unwarmed air to enter the bronchi. The condition occurs most frequently amongst elderly people, children and smokers of any age.

Bronchitis would be rare if people ate the right foods and their systems were not filled with mucus and poisonous waste matters, and if they wore proper clothing. Where there is bronchitis, there is usually stomach trouble or constipation. It is brought on by changeable weather, catching cold, exposure, wet feet, and chilling.

Bronchitis becomes chronic when acute bronchitis is not properly treated and relieved. When a cold is allowed to run, it gets down into the bronchial tubes and lungs and becomes chronic.

Clinical features of bronchitis

The initial symptom is an irritating, unproductive cough, accompanied by upper chest pain. As the bronchi become extensively involved, a sensation of tightness in the chest develops, and wheezing respiration and shortness of breath

59

may also occur. This group of symptoms is also sometimes termed as 'eosinophilia' or 'wheezy bronchitis'. Respiratory distress and shortness of breath may be particularly severe when acute bronchitis complicates underlying chronic bronchitis or emphysema.

Sputum is at first scanty, mucoid and difficult to bring up. Occasionally it may be streaked with blood. One or two days later it becomes thick and mucopurulent. As the inflammation descends down the bronchial tree, a moderate fever usually develops. Most cases recover over the next four to eight days without the patients ever becoming seriously ill.

Occasionally, the condition fails to resolve itself, and shortness of breath and other symptoms worsen, and fever continues to rise. This reflects that the body's vital resistance is lowered so that inflammation has continued into the alveoli and lungs themselves. The patient is then suffering from pneumonia and should be given high doses of antibiotics under a doctor's care.

Eosinophilia

Eosinophilia is a respiratory disorder with symptoms in common with both asthma and bronchitis and it is often difficult to decide which diagnostic label to assign to individual sufferers. The disorder is usually interpreted as a transition stage in respiratory diseases, when the sufferer from chronic cold or bronchitis is gradually evolving into a full-blown state of asthma. Eosinophilia is diagnosed when the percentage of eosinophils in the blood of the sufferer becomes elevated. Eosinophils are the white blood cells which mediate allergic and hypersensitive reactions, and an elevated level suggests that the asthma-like symptoms of the disease are an immune reaction by the lungs.

The cause of eosinophilia

The disorder is thought to be an allergic response to various foreign proteins and drugs, and in tropical countries it seems to appear as an allergic complication of filaria and worm infections. The disorder is common in industrial areas where air pollution is believed to be the major initiating factor. It is frequently diagnosed in children following investigation of persisting or recurrent cough and cold symptoms.

Medical management of chronic bronchitis and eosinophilia
Chronic or recurrent bronchial inflammation can be improved by making sure one has an adequate intake of fresh fruit and vegetables as well as sufficient vitamins and minerals for the body's metabolic needs. Fish oils have a strong anti-inflammatory effect when taken in therapeutic doses. Lastly, for the immune system to function at its optimum, the intake and digestion of proteins should be carefully monitored, as protein deficiency is a very common cause of suboptimal immune response. Appropriate physical exercise and deep breathing are aslso very useful.

Medical treatment of eosinophilia is far from effective. The drug diethylcarbamazine is prescribed where filarial infection is suspected, but this drug is minimally effective in the long term. Where drugs or medicines are likely initiating factors, they must be discontinued. Frequently the condition is indistinguishable from mild asthma.

Yogic management of chronic bronchitis and eosinophilia
Yoga therapy provides effective relief in cases of chronic bronchitis and eosinophilia and provides techniques for strengthening the weak and hypersensitive respiratory system. However, during an acute cough, cold or bronchitis, no asana should be practised at all and complete rest is necessary. Adopt the practice program gradually after the acute bout has subsided.

1. *Asana*: Commence with the pawanmuktasana series. Sufferers who are elderly or weak should practise only this series along with makarasana. Others are recommended to select a suitable practice program from amongst the following asanas in this order: Shakti bandha series, surya namaskara, vajrasana series (shashankasana,

shashank bhujangasana, ushtrasana, marjari-asana, supta vajrasana), pada hastasana, bhujangasana, dhanurasana, kandharasana, chakrasana, paschimottanasana, ardha matsyendrasana, baddha padmasana, sarvangasana, halasana and matsyasana.

Simhagarjanasana is especially recommended. Standing and bending asanas including trikonasana, hasta utthanasana, dwi konasana, lolasana, etc., will work to strengthen the chest.

2. *Pranayama*: All pranayama practices will enhance and develop the respiratory capacity and resistance. Especially recommended are ujjayi, kapalbhati, bhastrika and nadi shodhana (up to stage 3).

3. *Mudra and bandha*: Yoga mudra, prana mudra and maha bandha.

4. *Shatkarma*: Neti should be practised daily and kunjal should be performed daily for one week.

5. *Relaxation*: Yoga nidra provides deep relaxation and develops awareness. Often chronic cough becomes a characteristic habit and part of the personality of the sufferer from chronic bronchitis. In the beginning, the cough may worsen when yoga nidra is practised. This is usually a psychological reaction. One who has become accustomed to the habit of coughing does so unconsciously as a means of tension release. When all such activities and movements cease in yoga nidra, the psychological cough commonly asserts itself and the impulse to cough becomes prominent. The sufferer can evolve beyond this disease rapidly by recognizing the action of this coping mechanism in his or her lifestyle, and learn to resist and overcome it.

6. *Meditation*: Ajapa japa, with khechari mudra and ujjayi pranayama and rotating awareness from navel to throat and throat to navel in the frontal psychic passage, is also most valuable in helping to gradually recognize and relieve a chronic cough and respiratory weakness.

7. *Diet*: During an attack it is best to only take fruit and vegetable juices. Then barley water and watery khichari

or vegetable broth can be taken. Avoid cold drinks and foods. Eat plenty of vegetables, raw, steamed or lightly boiled. Citrus fruits help to loosen and cut the phlegm, as do onions, radishes and garlic. Hot milk with a little ginger and black pepper will also loosen the phlegm and facilitate its removal. This can be taken at night instead of the evening meal.

8. *Fasting*: This is highly recommended. If a full fast cannot be undertaken, it is advisable to miss the evening meal.

Further recommendations

- Avoid stuffy, overheated and unventilated rooms. Keep the chest and throat warm, but always ensure adequate ventilation, especially while sleeping. Avoid draughts and sitting on cold floors.
- Bronchitis sufferers should not take cold morning showers, and during the time of attacks, a hot steamy bath should be taken.
- Coughing should not be suppressed, as it is nature's way of clearing the phlegm and infective material from the bronchial tree. Removal of phlegm can be promoted by hot fomentations to the back and chest, then finishing with a cold fomentation.
- Smoking should be given up as it directly irritates the bronchial mucosa. Without giving up smoking, no measures will prove very effective in overcoming chronic bronchitis or eosinophilia.
- Daily walking is beneficial and deep breathing should be practised at intervals throughout the day.
- Steam inhalations at night are very helpful and hot foot baths with a tablespoon of mustard in the water.
- If a person is gasping for breath, rub the arms or feet hard in the direction of the heart.

Asthma

Asthma is a common and distressing condition which is characterized by recurrent attacks of spasm of the tubes of the lungs resulting in wheezing, coughing and a sense of suffocation. The larger airways (bronchi) constrict and become plugged with excessive, thick mucous secretions produced by the cells lining the airways.

Attacks of asthma may last for only a few minutes, or may continue for hours or even days, leaving the sufferer in a stage of physical, mental and emotional exhaustion. In rare and extreme cases, when the condition known as 'status asthmaticus' supervenes, asthma can even prove fatal.

The acute attack

An attack of asthma can be a fearful and exhausting experience for both the sufferer and their family members. The symptoms of an impending attack usually begin several hours prior to its actual onset and are, as a rule, constant and well recognized for each individual patient. They are commonly precipitated by bouts of emotional or psychological tension, by exercise, by dietary indiscretion, or by exposure to airborne allergens.

An impending attack in a child is often heralded by a slight wheeze, and a change in behaviour. The child may either become irritable and cry more readily, or become quiet, sluggish and introverted. Sometimes skin rashes may appear, and lips and face become swollen, indicating that the levels of emotional or immune stress are mounting to a level where crisis is imminent.

In most asthmatics there is a sudden onset of cold symptoms, such as nasal congestion, nasal irritation and bouts of sneezing, indicating that the nasal mucous membrane is becoming swollen and secretory in response to some psychological or environmental trigger. As the attack ensues, there is an increasing insufficiency of inhaled air (air hunger), causing great subjective distress and anxiety as respiration becomes more and more laboured. Mucus secretion becomes thick and sticky and a moist cough develops. The chest becomes hyperexpanded and the lungs hyperinflated. Expiration especially demands a continuous muscular effort in order to overcome the added resistance of thick sticky mucus plugging the respiratory tree. The patient may partially accomplish this by exhaling with pressed lips or while whistling, as this builds up the expiratory pressure in the lungs. As the attack continues, the colour of the mucous membranes may become bluish, which indicates that there is not enough oxygen entering the body.

An untreated attack usually continues in a vicious circle. The longer the sufferer fights to breathe, the longer the attack continues, and the more severe it becomes. The more severe the attack, the more distressed and anxious the sufferer becomes, and the less able to relax.

Long-term complications
The complications of asthma increase with the duration of the disease. The body becomes weak and debilitated. Asthmatic children commonly lag behind their peers in body weight and height. In addition, defects of posture, with permanent expansion of the ribcage and hunching of the shoulders, commonly accompany long-standing asthma.

The capacity to enjoy a fully active life and to participate in normal social and personal relationships is therefore reduced as the asthmatic is forced to lead an extremely sheltered life, with innumerable restrictions. Some asthmatics will have to take special medicines and avoid sports and other outdoor activities, and may derive secondary benefits by living up to the expectation of others and unconsciously fulfilling a sick, weak role. Thus the sufferer becomes increasingly entrapped in the web of illness and resistance to the disease diminishes.

The cause of asthma
The cause of asthma is multifactorial. Psychological, hereditary and allergic factors have all been implicated and are found to overlap variably from one patient to another. At the psychological level, suppression of negative emotions such as jealously, anger, resentment and hatred is often a precipitating cause, as are loneliness, longing for affection, emotional hypersensitivity, fear of rejection and hesitation in life. In management of asthma through yoga, these psychic factors are brought before the conscious mind. The sufferer learns to recognize, accept and gradually resolve these difficulties.

Asthma can arise at any age, but it is especially common in children and adolescents. Its onset may be gradual or sudden. Asthmatics often report that the disease developed soon after the some loss, rejection or major threat to personal security. Examples include the loss of a parent, child, partner or important job opportunity.

Another causative factor is exposure to allergens, that is, substances causing heightened sensitivity. These may be food products, drugs, medicine, different types of dust, animal hair, environmental and atmospheric pollution.

Asthma can also arise during changing climatic conditions, and incidence of attacks is higher in the winter and rainy season in the tropics. Bouts of sneezing, hay fever, 'wheezy bronchitis' or eosinophilia may progress towards overt asthma over a period of time. Eosinophilia is really a stage of pre-asthma and shows that the body's self-defence system is being aroused against an irritant, either some psychic threat or fear-inducing factor, or increased exposure to some physical allergen, like industrial smoke or diesel fumes.

Unhealthy diet and lifestyle also play a role in the genesis of asthma. A low residue, mucus producing diet consisting of excessive refined carbohydrate products like bread and cakes, ghee, oily preparations, milk and milk products, while deficient in fruits, vegetables and unrefined grains, is commonly incriminated. Besides producing mucus, this diet is excessively taxing on the asthmatic's pre-weakened digestive processes.

The hereditary factor in asthma is also well recognized, for the disease frequently appears to be passed on from one generation to another within a family. Even where no positive family history of asthma is detected, there is often a family tendency to some other hypersensitivity, allergic or psychosomatic disorder such as eczema. It is a disease of low energy which is frequently observed to develop secondary to digestive weakness, where intestinal sluggishness and constipation have become chronic problems.

Psychological factors

Generally the asthmatic is one who has undergone some form of painful rejection or loss early in life, which he has been unable to accept subconsciously, even if his conscious mind has come to terms with it. For example, a young child who has been deprived of his mother and left alone to confront the world can learn to trust no one but himself, for he finds no solace or wisdom in trusting the natural order that has dealt him such an unacceptable and painful blow. As a result, he may grow up excessively sensitive to what is his, for he fears that again he will mercilessly lose his most valuable possession.

A small child deprived of the enormous security of his mother feels deprived of any reality. He clutches at anything which will give his life meaning and so it is that he begins to clutch for his breath at times when he feels threatened, either by psychological or environmental agents. Paradoxically, the more anxious he becomes, the more he clutches for his breath, and the more elusive it becomes. This is an emotional ordeal as well as a physical one. The sufferer feels he is all alone without anyone to depend on, fighting for his very existence, as symbolized by his elusive breath.

For a complete cure of asthma it is necessary to open the heart, express the emotions and develop trust.

The role of drugs
Medical science has developed a range of powerful drugs which effectively avert the symptoms of an acute attack, and also decrease the incidence of attacks. However, they do not cure the condition and may make the sufferer weaker and sicker. They also create psychological and, in some cases, physiological dependence. Most asthmatics have a great fear of being forced to confront an attack without resort to drugs.

In yoga therapy, the first step is to give sufferers the experience of successfully managing the condition using yoga techniques along with recourse to medicine only when it is absolutely necessary. As confidence in their own abilities to avert and control the symptoms of an attack increases, they are able to gradually discontinue the drugs and medications upon which they are depending.

Anti-asthma drugs should not be discontinued suddenly without proper guidance, as this often allows asthma previously suppressed by drugs to 'bounce back'. It is best accomplished in a hospital or yogic ashram, especially when the patient is depending on drugs such as cortisone, which not only suppress the body's own hormonal capacities and create physiological addiction, but also have severe side effects. These drugs should be avoided in all but the most severe cases.

Nutritional management of asthma
The main pathological changes in asthma consist of inflammation of the bronchial lining and spasm of the smooth muscle surrounding the bronchi. There is good

clinical evidence that addressing both these issues will help to diminish the severity and frequency of attacks. Inflammation can be worsened by poor immune function, exposure to allergenic food and deficiency of anti-inflammatory nutrients. These include vitamin C, the B complex, zinc, calcium, vitamin D3 and quercetin. Another key anti-inflammatory substance is omega-3 fatty acids, ideally derived from oily cold-water fish, such as tuna, sardines as well as cod liver oil and flaxseed oil.

To lessen the degree of bronchospasm, increase the intake of magnesium.

Yogic management of asthma

An essential part of yogic management is restoration of depleted and blocked pranic energy channels. This is achieved gradually by the combined influence of yogasana, pranayama and shatkarma. These should be learned during a residential stay in an ashram and practised with determination. Only with consistent and regular daily practice is complete and lasting drug free recovery possible. In this way, cure of asthma in the shortest time, with the minimal amount of suffering will be attained.

It is not possible to attain lasting relief or cure in an asthmatic in whom constipation remains. In seeking to cure the disorder in these cases, it is first necessary to remove constipation and to increase digestive heat in the body. In this way the inherent low energy tendency which predisposes a person to asthma can be overcome. Constipation is not only a condition of the intestines, but also of the mind. Its relief brings about a welcome release of previously bound up mental and emotional energy. The following practices relieve constipation from the bowels, lungs and mind.

1. *Surya namaskara*: Perform it slowly and with breath awareness. Practise up to 7 rounds each morning at sunrise.
2. *Asana*: Those whose bodies are stiff should first practise the pawanmuktasana series for a few weeks. Then commence some of the following:

69

Hasta utthanasana, dwi konasana, marjari-asana, shashank bhujangasana, dhanurasana, pranamasana, kandharasana, makarasana, gomukhasana, sarvangasana, matsyasana, simhagarjanasana, baddha padmasana, lolasana, tolangulasana, parivritti janu sirshasana. These asanas help to reshape the chest, improve posture, strengthen the spinal column, promote the flow of inhibited and blocked nervous energy, and rebalance and restore the whole body. Practise all the asanas with full awareness of the breath as well as the body.

3. *Pranayama*: This is important in averting acute attacks by strengthening the entire nervous system, restoring balance to a depleted and imbalanced autonomic nervous system and enhancing voluntary control over the respiratory mechanisms. Nadi shodhana develops awareness and control over the inflowing and outflowing breath. Bhastrika, with both kumbhaka and jalandhara bandha, strengthens the lungs and improves respiratory capacity. With regular practice of pranayama, the asthmatic learns to be more and more aware of the breath and, automatically becomes aware of thoughts, feelings and mental states.

4. *Shatkarma*: These are the most important part of the therapy. Warm saline water is profoundly effective in dissolving and removing thickened accumulated mucous wastes from the nasal mucous membranes, the respiratory tree, the stomach and the lower digestive tract. Kunjal and neti should be performed each morning before any other sadhana.

By practising kunjal kriya, an acute attack of asthma can be terminated and a threatened attack can be averted by directing the build-up of nervous energy that is causing the attack, towards expelling the water from the stomach. Nervous spasm and tension in the smooth muscles of the respiratory tree are released by the reflex action of the vagus nerve. Vastra dhauti is also an excellent practice, but it should only be attempted under expert guidance.

Neti kriya removes obstructions from the nasal passages, facilitates nasal breathing and averts the allergic and hypersensitivity responses mediated through the nasal mucous membrane and its autonomic nervous connections, precipitating bouts of asthma.

Shankhaprakshalana is vital in restoring the asthmatic's depleted digestive energy and in eliminating constipation. The full form is time-consuming and tiring and should only be performed once under guidance in an ashram at the commencement of therapy. Laghoo shankhaprakshalana can be practised each alternate morning for a week and then repeated whenever there is constipation.

5. *Relaxation*: Yoga nidra provides an effective means for defusing an acute attack of asthma. It is also useful in inducing the state of mental relaxation in which yogic self-analysis can occur. Practise it daily, and if there is insufficient time for the full technique, practise abdominal breath awareness in shavasana. This will enable the asthmatic to become familiar with his or her estranged breathing process.

6. *Meditation*: Ajapa japa, ascending and descending the consciousness in the frontal psychic passageway from the navel to the throat in conjunction with the mantra *So-ham*. The practice slows and releases the breath, allowing the deeper subconscious psychic factors which initiate and underlie asthma to surface. It is an essential part of the cure that an asthmatic learns to recognize and accept what has been suppressed for so long.

7. *Diet*: Simple, nourishing, non-stimulating foods, including plenty of fresh fruit and lightly cooked vegetables, particularly greens. Take wholemeal grains and pulses in place of meat and eggs. Mucus forming foods such as rice, sweets, dairy products and refined flour products should be completely avoided. Heavy, oily and dried foods should not be taken as they excessively tax the already weakened digestive energy. All chemically treated, processed, flavoured and preserved foods, as well as any foods which are known to initiate an allergic reaction, should be strictly avoided.

It is best to have the heavier meal at lunch time and a small light meal in the evening. It is good to take fruit juice or fruit only for breakfast or to take nothing but fruit for a few days.

Heating spices such as chilli, pepper, garlic and ginger are recommended, especially in the colder months when *kapha* (the mucous element) increases in the body.

8. *Fasting*: If a full fast cannot be undertaken, it is a good habit to miss the evening meal and take only hot lemon juice and honey, herbal tea (lemon grass, tulsi, ginger, black pepper) or a special preparation of karha can be prepared by boiling together heating spices (ginger, black pepper, cinnamon, cardamon, tulsi and vanfasa). This mixture is prepared by boiling away half the liquid on a simmering fire. Honey can then be added just before drinking.

Further recommendations

• As soon as an attack appears to be imminent, instead of reaching for drugs, the asthmatic should perform kunjal kriya or, in the case where a meal has recently been eaten, vyaghra kriya. This should be followed by neti and the practice of abdominal breathing in shavasana. This provides a means of maintaining union between the mind and breath, so that alienation or separation from the breath, which is the basic psychic experience of the asthmatic during the attack, is avoided.

• Physical fitness should be developed and excess weight removed, as it accentuates the respiratory difficulties of an asthmatic. Swimming provides excellent exercise for asthmatics. Running and jogging are also useful in moderation. Never perform them competitively, but use them as a means of developing spontaneous breath and mantra awareness.

• A cold shower should be taken every morning, paying particular attention to apply cold water to the neck and shoulders.

• An effective remedy can be made by laying very thin slices of raw onion and garlic on a plate and spreading honey on each slice. Cover with an inverted plate and let it stand all night. Take a spoonful of the resultant syrup four times a day.

Sinusitis and Hay Fever

Sinusitis and hay fever are troublesome conditions which tend to recur each spring or monsoon season in susceptible individuals. Medical scientists view these upper respiratory tract disorders as being caused by viruses or defects in our immune system. The underlying cause is recognized by yogic science as an excess of the mucous element in the body.

Sinusitis

Sinusitis is a state of inflammation of the sinus cavities in the cheeks and frontal bones. These cavities, which are lined by mucous membrane, open into the nasal passages. During a bout of cold, the narrow entrances into the sinuses become blocked, and headache and stuffiness are experienced, together with swelling and tenderness over the cheek bones and forehead. Sometimes, pain in the sinuses can become very severe and it can be accompanied by aching in the eyes. However, these symptoms should clear up together with the cold within a week, given rest and proper care.

Chronic sinusitis

Sinusitis may become a chronic condition lasting for two weeks, a month, or even more. This usually occurs when an acute cold is neglected, wrong eating habits continue and auto-intoxication develops due to constipation. As a result, bacterial infection, production of mucopurulent sputum and descent of symptoms into the lower respiratory tract (bronchitis) occurs. Facial swelling and bone tenderness usually pass off, but a persistent mucopurulent discharge into the front and back of the nose from the congested, infected sinuses, accompanied by nasal obstruction and recurrent headaches, become the prominent symptoms.

In chronic sinusitis, a deep-seated infection has become established which proves extremely difficult and troublesome to overcome by conventional medical measures. Apart from problems of reinfection, chronic sinusitis serves as a constant source for other respiratory diseases.

Nervous stress and emotional upset also have a prominent role in persistent sinusitis, chronic cold and recurring headaches. Physicians note that sneezing attacks and nasal irritation often accompany periods of emotional upset. Sinus troubles of this kind respond rapidly to yogic therapy.

Hay fever (allergic rhinitis)

Hay fever is closely related to sinusitis. It typically comes on suddenly, and at about the same time every year. There is a tickling in the nose, sneezing and irritation down into the bronchial tubes. Symptoms are like those of a cold but more severe. The eyes are filled with tears and there is acute swelling and irritation of the nasal mucous membrane and sinuses, profuse mucus discharge and headache.

Medical scientists classify hay fever as an allergy which may develop following exposure to some inhaled irritant such as pollen or house dust, or it may be precipitated by an allergen taken in the diet. Chocolate, milk, bananas, strawberries and and oranges are some of the substances known to precipitate hay fever in affected individuals. However, according to yogic understanding, when the digestive organs and the nasal membranes are in good health such irritants cannot affect us.

Hay fever occurs due to hypersensitivity of the individual's immune surveillance system, perhaps due to sensitization to

74

the offending allergen in the past. When the individual comes into contact with the allergen, a violent inflammatory reaction is set into motion, precipitated by the release of the chemical histamine into the bloodstream.

Often the hypersensitivity can be traced back to traumatic events and experiences which generated deep subconscious, negative influences and associations in childhood. Because the priming of the immune system and the laying down of subconscious impressions occur simultaneously throughout life, especially during childhood, it is often extremely difficult to separate allergic from psychological components in sinusitis, hay fever and asthma. Psychological programming and immune sensitization are like two sides of a single coin, and the immune system of an adult seems to be a kind of cellular memory of our experiences.

Yogic science explains hypersensitive reactions as the arousal of a previously developed mental samskara, or impression, which has left a deep-set memory and imprint in both our psyche and cellular memory (surveillance system). The person who suddenly starts sneezing either in a tense psychological situation or when exposed to house dust is manifesting essentially the same reaction. It is a physiological immune response to a subconscious mental impression surfacing.

Medical management of sinusitis and hay fever

Medical management of sinusitis and hay fever normally consists of analgesics for pain relief, anti-histamines to suppress allergic reactions and antibiotics to protect against secondary infections. Some of these drugs have adverse side-effects, such as the drowsiness produced by anti-histamines, and none of them has any effect on the root causes of the problem.

Until recently, courses of desensitizing injections to dull the body's increased sensitivity to specific irritants and allergens were a popular treatment for allergies in children. They have, however, fallen into disfavour with many medical practitioners because they are expensive, require many painful injections and rarely provide the immunity to allergens that was originally expected. There is also an increasing awareness of the dangers of precipitating more severe immune disorders, hypersensitivity states and even cancers, by injecting foreign materials into the bloodstream.

In severe chronic sinusitis, the surgical procedure of antral washout is sometimes performed. By piercing the bony wall of a blocked and painful sinus, saline water can be introduced into the seat of chronic inflammation in the sinus, and total washing and evacuation can be performed. This is a painful, time-consuming surgical procedure which gives only transient relief. The yogic practice of neti is far better from both the doctor's and patient's viewpoints as it is cheap, easy and enjoyable and provides better long-term results.

Nutritional management of sinusitis and hay fever

It is essential to have good hydration and a diet high in omega-3 essential fatty acids (i.e. fish, almonds, walnuts, pumpkin and flax seeds), onions, fruits and vegetables (at least five servings a day). A number of supplements are also helpful, including vitamin C (at least 2 gm/day), quercetin, bromelain, vitamin A and garlic.

Yogic management of sinusitis and hay fever

The cure of sinusitis and hay fever can be achieved in two ways: by balancing the body's energy systems or nadis, and by throwing light upon the deeper mental impressions and blockages which arise simultaneously with the symptoms. Meditation, yoga nidra and objective self-analysis frequently enable the unconscious mechanism of these conditions to be understood and transcended.

In general, asanas are contraindicated in febrile conditions but can be adopted after fever and other debilitating symptoms have diminished.

1. *Surya namaskara*: This dynamic practice dramatically raises the level of pranic energy in the body, counteracts

excessive cold and overcomes many psychological and immune deficiencies and hypersensitive states. It helps to throw off resistant respiratory infections.

2. *Asana*: Pawanmuktasana is the best series to commence with in the recovery period. Follow with surya namaskara and shavasana, as strength improves, then paschimottanasana, bhujangasana, halasana, dhanurasana and ardha matsyendrasana can be practised one to three times each according to capacity. Simhagarjanasana should also be practised.

Sirshasana and sarvangasana are contraindicated when there are symptoms of cold as they may precipitate sinusitis or complicate an existing case of sinusitis.

3. *Pranayama*: Bhastrika, up to 5 rounds of 50 breaths.

4. *Shatkarma*: Jala neti is most beneficial provided there is no fever. It removes nasal mucus, drains and aerates the sinuses. Practise once or twice daily, or whenever relief of stuffiness and mucus build-up is required. Immediately after jala neti, perform kapalbhati to clear and dry the nasal passages and activate the frontal area of the brain. Unless all excess water is removed from the nose, neti may have detrimental effects, including initiation of further colds.

Sutra neti is an effective practice to desensitize the nasal mucous membranes. In the first few days the practice may provoke sneezing and irritation, but it will get easier with practice.

Kunjal kriya is very beneficial in both prevention and treatment and can be practised daily. Shankhaprakshalana should be performed at each change of season to remove decaying mucus wastes from the digestive system and reset the body thermostat.

5. *Relaxation*: Yoga nidra should be practised daily as it is deeply relaxing and highly therapeutic. It enables the hay fever or sinusitis sufferer to witness the underlying personal complexes and perceptions arising from the past conditioning and prior childhood experiences, which so frequently initiate these diseases.

6. *Diet*: A light, non-mucous forming vegetarian diet should be followed. Avoid overeating, especially heavy, oily and sweet foods, and abstain from salt, rice and refined flour products. Eat plenty of fruit and raw vegetables. A fruit juice diet for three or four days is highly recommended. Drink plenty of citrus or grape juice, but do not mix the juices. After this, include plenty of vegetables in the diet and continue to eat lots of fruit, particularly papaya. Avoid taking cold or iced drinks, milk, ice cream and other dairy products. Take some fresh garlic every day.

7. *Fasting*: Fast whenever symptoms appear to be increasing. This is a most effective means of avoiding attacks. Alternatively, substitute the evening meal each day with tea prepared from substances such as ginger, pepper, cinnamon and cardamon, which heat the body and promote mucus elimination.

Further recommendations

- Keep the body warm in the winter and monsoon seasons. Particularly make sure that the neck and chest are protected from the cold.
- Take complete rest as soon as symptoms of hay fever or sinusitis appear, avoid baths and don't drink too much water.
- A special preparation can be made for neti. Make a solution using a rounded teaspoonful of golden seal, or turmeric, a little salt and a heaped teaspoonful of borax in a pint of boiling water. Shake well. Let it stand for an hour or two shaking occasionally. Then use it in the neti lota. Repeat until the nose is entirely clean. This is very healing and soothing to the mucous membrane and should be done three times a day. It is often beneficial to use urine neti.
- Cold applications over the sinuses or alternate hot and cold applications will give relief.
- Steam inhalations at night will ease symptoms.
- Smoking should be discontinued.

Tonsillitis

The tonsils are two areas of sensitive immune tissue lying on either side of the pharynx, at the entrance to the throat. These glandular structures form the first line of defence of the body's immune surveillance system, being part of a larger circle of protective lymphoid tissue called the Waldeyer's Ring, which also includes the adenoids. They stand guard like twin sentries protecting the body from invasion by micro-organisms, such as bacteria and viruses, and are also responsible for recognizing and responding to potential allergens and any foreign substances, foods and chemicals.

Tonsillitis

Tonsillitis means inflammation of the tonsils, which become red, swollen, tender and may be covered with creamy white pus and decaying material. This disorder of children and adolescents usually recurs at intervals during growth and development as the immune system is exposed to new micro-organisms and other environmental substances. Tonsillar inflammation frequently precedes severe systemic infections and may precede serious diseases such as rheumatic heart disease, arthritis and kidney disease. Generalized febrile states and conditions such as constipation may also precipitate tonsillitis, as well as other immune and lymphatic tissue responses including appendicitis and lymphadenitis.

Bouts of tonsillitis are often precipitated by dietary abuse in susceptible individuals. Cold foods and drinks are especially implicated. Exposure of the body to wet and cold conditions is another frequent precipitating factor.

The onset of tonsillitis is preceded by chilly feelings and pains in the back and limbs. Fever rises rapidly and in young children may reach 105 degrees on the evening of the first day. Sore throat and difficulty in swallowing are prominent. The breath becomes heavy and foul and the tongue becomes furred. The voice often becomes nasal and swelling of the cervical lymph glands in the side of the neck is common. Generally fever departs within a week and inflammation gradually subsides, but the tonsils often remain swollen.

Chronic tonsillitis

Chronic tonsillitis is long-term enlargement of the tonsils. It occurs in children and young adults, and is usually associated with swelling of the adenoids, a second smaller group of lymphatic glands in the pharynx.

The habit of breathing through the mouth due to chronic inflammation of the tonsils and adenoids is perhaps the most far-reaching effect because it is found to adversely affect subsequent physical and mental development. Deformation of the chest, changes in facial expression, alteration of mental condition and stunting of growth are characteristic features of children who become mouth breathers. The face may assume a characteristic vacant, dull and apathetic expression, especially in sleep. Weakening of mental capacities and memory and slowing down of the thought processes are further consequences.

These major detrimental effects of mouth breathing reveal the importance of a free and balanced flow of breath through both nostrils in healthy physical and mental development, and give us some glimpse of the therapeutic value of pranayama practices such as nadi shodhana and kapalbhati, as well as jala and sutra neti kriyas.

Yogic physiology

According to yogic physiology, the nostrils are the roots of the two major nadis in the psychic body known as ida and pingala. Ida nadi conducts *chitta shakti* (mental energy), responsible for mental development and expression. Pingala nadi conducts *prana shakti* (vital energy), responsible for physical action and development. Balance of physical and mental capacities and energies is achieved in hatha yoga and pranayama by balancing and equalizing the flow of breath in the nostrils, and this leads to full development and awakening of the dormant mental and physical capacities of the individual.

Physiological discoveries closely augment the yogic contentions. A vast number of autonomic and sensory nerves are found to lie closely exposed beneath the nasal mucous membrane, and these are differentially stimulated by the twin flows of breath in the nostrils, producing widespread physical and mental effects. The importance of arresting chronic tonsillitis, adenoid inflammation, habitual mouth breathing and nasal deviations and deformities is clearly paramount in the future health, well-being and mental development of the afflicted child or adolescent.

Medical management

Medical management of chronic tonsillitis in the past was usually by surgical removal, termed tonsillectomy. In more recent times the frequency of this operation has fallen dramatically as doctors have become more aware of the long-term dangers of surgical removal of vital organs from the immune system. There is mounting evidence that the likelihood of more severe lymphatic or immune system diseases and infections is increased in those who have undergone surgical removal of the tonsils (tonsillectomy). Certainly modern surgeons are more reticent to remove major lymphatic glandular structures such as the appendix and tonsils, than they used to be. This reflects the growing understanding of the role of these lymphatic structures in health and disease.

81

Antibiotics usually play a prominent role in the medical management of tonsillitis. Courses of antibiotics are often prescribed to quell troublesome recurrences of the symptoms with every change of season. However, cure of tonsillitis by this method is rare.

Acute tonsillitis may be seen as the manifestation of underlying physical imbalance and impurity rather than sickness. When the acute attack is over, instead of taking the tonsils out, use yoga to cleanse and rebalance the body.

Note: Many sufferers from recurrent or chronic tonsillitis have an impaired immune system, which is often exacerbated by an underlying intolerance to dairy products. A trial of dairy-free diet for three to six months could be diagnostic as well as therapeutic.

Yogic management of chronic sore throat, tonsillitis and mouth breathing

Yogic techniques provide safe and effective relief of chronic tonsillitis. Correction of habitual mouth breathing can also be attained by regular and persistent practice of the following program. In acute tonsillitis with fever, rest in bed until the temperature and acute phase of the illness subsides. Antibiotic therapy may also be required along with an analgesic such as aspirin, during the initial attack. Relief will also be gained by saline gargling, neti and hot fomentations on the neck region. After the acute bout subsides, the following yoga program should be adopted, according to capability.

1. *Surya namaskara*: Practise to capacity with full awareness of the breath.
2. *Asana*: Simhagarjanasana, balancing asanas, trikonasana.
3. *Pranayama*: Ujjayi, sheetali, seetkari and nadi shodhana.
4. *Shatkarma*: Neti and gargling with warm salty water twice a day, kunjal and laghoo shankhaprakshalana as required.
5. *Relaxation*: Yoga nidra.
6. *Diet*: In the acute phase take only fruit juice and mung sprouts mixed with a little oil, lemon juice and crushed garlic. Then take vegetable broth and light khichari.

Further recommendations

- The throat should be kept warm at all times. Exposure to cold outside air during an attack is harmful as the moisture and dust in the air inflame the tonsils.
- If the tonsils are very swollen and painful, crush some ice. Wrap it in a towel and put it around the neck. When this becomes uncomfortable, take it off and apply a hot fomentation. Keep it on for three to five minutes. Then put the ice on again. Keep this up for half an hour, then gargle with warm salty water.
- Gargling with warm salty water or an antiseptic mouthwash twice a day brings relief and promotes healing.

Gastro-Intestinal Tract

Disorders of the
Digestive System

Many people today are depriving themselves of one of the most simple yet profound pleasures of life, the possession of a healthy digestive and eliminative system. It is fundamental to the enjoyment of life, as our digestion influences our whole perception and appreciation of life. The intimate relationship between the functioning of the mind and body has now become widely accepted in all forms of healing.

A healthy digestive and eliminative system is absolutely fundamental to good physical and mental health. A vast number of chronic degenerative and metabolic diseases are secondary effects of long-term malfunctions and abuse of the digestive system. In these diseases we include asthma, diabetes, arthritis, heart and vascular disorders, skin diseases, cancers, headaches, mental diseases, sexual disorders and other endocrine malfunctions. These debilitating and often fatal processes have their genesis in disturbed digestion, assimilation and elimination.

Therefore, in attempting to ameliorate or manage major diseases, it is frequently necessary to initially rebalance and strengthen the primary digestive processes, because if the shakti or vital energy can be awakened and balanced, then regenerative processes are set in motion automatically and self-healing will spontaneously begin. Activating the body's inherent healing energy is a fundamental principle of yogic management.

The role of digestive power

To maintain optimal health and vitality in life, it is necessary that we develop a most subtle yet important capacity which most people lack, and which leads them to much suffering, discomfort and disease. We all have to know how to eat. This means that we have to know how to maintain our physical body in a state of health and high vital resistance by taking in only the right foods in only the necessary quantities at only the correct times. This sounds so simple, but it is a rare person indeed who has understood and mastered its implications.

Most diseases result, either directly or indirectly, from having failed to learn this great lesson. From the point of view of our physical health, whenever we use the eating mechanism for other purposes, such as the satisfaction of emotional needs, to relieve frustration, as an outlet for greed and so on, we are using it wrongly and have commenced to travel the road to sickness, disease and physical decay which first manifests as digestive disturbance.

Manipura chakra

In kundalini yoga, the digestive organs, glands and the solar plexus of nerves are symbolized by manipura chakra. Its element is fire and its symbol is the blazing orb of the sun. Just as the external sun is the source of life, energy and heat in our solar system, so our physical body and its metabolic processes are maintained by a healthy digestive fire, a blazing inner sun.

We can consider the digestive process to be a fire into which fuel, the products of the earth, are fed and which is fanned from above by the bellows of the diaphragm and the air element (anahata chakra) governing the heart and respiratory system. It is supported by the water element (swadhisthana chakra), which governs the elimination of liquid wastes by the kidneys and sweat glands. The whole process is grounded in the earth element (mooladhara – the base chakra in the perineum), to which the solid wastes of the digestive process are returned. Thus we have a sound model for our consideration of digestive disorders.

The gastro-intestinal tract

The best way to consider the digestive system is as a hollow tube or pipe which has two openings: the upper opening at the mouth and the lower opening at the anus. Food is placed in one end and the wastes are expelled at the other. In between, the processes of digestion, absorption and assimilation of nutrients into our physical frame, as well as elimination of toxic and unabsorbed waste products occurs.

The gastro-intestinal tract can be conveniently divided into three divisions: upper, middle and lower digestive tracts. We will outline the disorders of each in this chapter and then discuss them individually in the subsequent chapters.

The upper digestive tract

The upper digestive tract includes the mouth and salivary glands, the oesophagus and the stomach, which are considered in yogic physiology to be essentially under the control of prana, the first of the five pranic subdivisions. This force operates from the throat down to the diaphragm, and from the diaphragm up to the throat.

Upper digestive tract disorders are essentially due to imbalance between the air and fire elements. They include hyperacidity and hypoacidity, gastritis and peptic ulcer, and give rise to many common symptoms, including belching, wind, heartburn and indigestion, reflux and regurgitation.

The middle digestive tract

The middle digestive tract is the segment extending from the duodenum down to the termination of the small intestine (iliocecal valve) where the lower eliminative segment, known as the colon or large intestine, begins. The mid-digestive tract is responsible for absorption and assimilation of digested matter into the bloodstream. The division of prana responsible for this central assimilation process is termed samana. It circulates between the navel and the heart and controls the body's metabolic rate and temperature.

The middle digestive tract is comprised of three major organs – the liver, the small intestine (ileum) and the pancreas. Disorders of the mid-digestive tract therefore include diseases of the liver, gastro-enteritis, malabsorption states and diabetes.

The lower digestive tract

The lower digestive tract begins at the termination of the small intestine in the ileocecal valve. Beyond this valve, the large intestine or colon begins. The descending liquid matter being propelled along the tract is now considered as waste material, as all nutrients were extracted during its passage through the small intestine. The division of prana which sustains the operation of the lower digestive tract is known as apana. This prana flows downwards from the navel region to the perineum and it is responsible for the expulsion of faecal matter and urine from the body.

Excesses and deficiencies of apana lead to abnormal lower digestive function, and many acute and chronic diseases stem directly from this fundamental source. They include constipation, diarrhoea, haemorrhoids, dysentery, appendicitis, colitis, diverticulitis and prolapse.

Hatha yoga

The yogis who foresaw the coming need for yoga also realized the importance of the digestive tract and dedicated a large part of their preliminary practices to cleansing and maintaining good abdominal health. Asanas, some pranayamas and shatkarmas, including dhauti, nauli and basti, aim to purify and heal the digestive tract as well as other body systems. These techniques transform the digestive tract from being purely a food processing plant into the source for our ascent into higher awareness and a more creative, fuller life.

Complete information is contained in *The Practices of Yoga for the Digestive System*, published by Yoga Publications Trust.

The Upper Digestive Disorders

The wide range of malfunctions in the upper digestive system stem from indigestion, a general term that includes the states of excessive acid production and motility of the stomach (hyperacidity) which occur in peptic ulcer and gastritis, and also the opposite extreme of diminished gastric activity and secretion (hypoacidity), such as occurs in reflux and regurgitation. Both extremes are characterized by failure of synchronization of secretory and motile functions of the stomach, termed dyspepsia.

The cause of indigestion

The various digestive diseases have a multitude of causes including mental and emotional disturbance, the habit of swallowing air and gluttony. Other prime causes of indigestion or dyspepsia are a diet deficient in mineral salts, eating too many refined foods such as those made of white flour and cane sugar, drinking with meals, hasty or irregular meals, late suppers, highly seasoned foods, poor mastication and iced drinks. The result is that the digestive system is weakened and the sufferer cannot digest the foods which would repair the deficiency.

Signs and symptoms

The symptoms which generally indicate indigestion are heartburn, headache, heaviness in the stomach, irregularity

91

of the bowels, cold feet, weak pulse and, in chronic cases, general prostration. In long-standing cases there will be a hacking cough, intermittent fever, palpitation of the heart and irritability.

Specific disorders

Hypoacidity is a state where food remains fermenting in the stomach for several hours after it has been eaten, and represents a failure of digestive power. There are inadequate salivary enzymes and an insufficient amount of gastric acid to continue active digestion, so the whole process comes to a standstill. Food is felt to sit in the stomach for hours, and the stomach may still be full three to four hours after the last meal. Vyaghra kriya is highly recommended.

Hypoacidity is usually an indication that food in excess of body requirements and capacities is being consumed. It may occur due to long-term liver and intestinal abuse and exhaustion, and occurs to some extent in most people in the hot summer and monsoon months, when dietary discretion becomes essential.

Regurgitation is when liquid, partially digested food materials from the stomach rise back up the oesophagus and into the throat. In the hours after eating, sensations of nausea, together with the unpleasant sensation that digestion is not proceeding satisfactorily, accompany hypoacidity.

Hyperacidity is the other extreme, where the digestive processes are constantly overactivated, with untimely secretion and pooling of gastric acids in a churning, activated stomach, even when it remains empty of food contents. This is the situation which leads to the development of gastritis and peptic ulcer.

The fundamental cause of hyperacidity is constant over-stimulation of the taste buds and salivary glands, which in turn causes constant stimulation of digestive activity in the stomach. This occurs through addiction to an imbalanced diet which is selected purely on the basis of taste and oral satisfaction, rather than with regard for its suitability and health promoting qualities. A diet full of sugar, condiments, sweets, refined and excessively rich, spicy and pungent foods is usually incriminated, and is worsened by oral addictions such as drinking alcohol and smoking.

These 'tasty' foods and compulsive habits provide oral satisfaction, temporarily relieving a state of tension and anxiety due to emotional frustration. Habits of smoking, drinking and eating excessively rich foods, to provide oral satisfaction lead to a state of constant gastric secretion and churning of the stomach, irrespective of whether food is present or not. They are the most common precipitators of hyperacidity, gastritis and peptic ulcers.

According to psychologists, this problem stems from an experience in infancy, when the individual was deprived of the security of the mother's breast as the source of both dietary and emotional satisfaction. As a result, there is an unresolved frustration, with the constant need to have some form of oral satisfaction as a source of emotional security in adult life.

Heartburn refers to the symptom of burning irritation and pain which accompanies hyperacidity, and is due to acid irritation of the lower end of the oesophagus. This painful sensation is experienced directly behind the sternum in the centre of the chest. It occurs after eating, and may be confused initially with the clasping chest pain caused by coronary insufficiency (cardiac angina) which may also follow a heavy meal.

Wind refers to the sensation of fullness or bloating in the upper abdomen which occurs whenever food is eaten hurriedly, without awareness, or in incorrect combinations. When food is gulped down quickly and carelessly, while the body or mind remain anxious and preoccupied, air is swallowed unconsciously along with the food, which is not chewed and masticated properly. Rapid, anxious eating can become a habit, and frequently leads to hyperacidity and wind formation. There is often an awareness of enhanced stomach movement and noises, with marked upper abdominal swelling and discomfort.

Belching, or burping, is a closely related symptom referring to the expulsion of wind from the stomach. Gas rises up into the oesophagus and is expelled from the mouth. A degree of belching is a necessary and desirable accompaniment of successful digestion as the stomach churns its contents again and again. However, where excessive air has been swallowed due to hasty consumption of overly rich food, belching becomes excessive and troublesome in the hours following the meal. Symptoms of wind and belching usually accompany hypoacidity.

The solution to digestive problems
The importance of elevating the eating process from a mechanical habit to a conscious and pleasurable act in which a moderate quantity of simple, pure food, sufficient to maintain the body's requirements, is eaten with full awareness, cannot be overestimated. By cultivating this ability, habits of overeating, hasty eating and eating overly rich foods are slowly but surely eradicated from the lifestyle, and better general health and vitality are rapidly gained.

The two extremes of indigestion – hypoacidity and hyperacidity, may occur in isolation in particular sufferers. More frequently, the two extremes follow one another cyclically according to the seasons, in people who suffer from uncontrolled eating habits and unsuitable diets, especially in hot or extreme climates. In these cases there is often a digestive imbalance which demands correction through yogic and dietary measures if more serious harm to the overall state of physical health is to be avoided.

Yogic management of indigestion
The following practices are specific for upper digestive disorders and will restore function rapidly if practised daily.
1. *Asana*: Pawanmuktasana series part 2, the antigastric exercises, should be practised each morning. Vajrasana should be adopted for ten minutes immediately after each meal. This posture promotes optimal digestion.

2. *Pranayama*: Nadi shodhana stage 2, 10 rounds each morning. Then progress to stage 3. Bhastrika should also be practised; gradually build up to 5 rounds of 50 breaths.
3. *Bandha*: Jalandhara, moola and uddiyana should be incorporated into pranayama practices.
4. *Shatkarma*: Neti, kunjal, vyaghra kriya and agnisar kriya. Laghoo shankhaprakshalana should be practised for at least a week.
5. *Relaxation*: Practise yoga nidra each afternoon or evening. After asana, relax in shavasana and practise 100 abdominal or yogic respirations.
6. *Meditation*: Sit in padmasana or vajrasana and concentrate on the movement of breath at the navel.
7. *Diet*: Simple, nourishing and easily digestible foods are best. Avoid spicy, rich and pungent preparations, cakes, refined flour products, sweets, , which are a burden to the stomach and promote over-production of acid. The diet should consist of freshly prepared natural foods, with simple boiled or steamed vegetables, coarse chapatis, rice, salads, fruit and pulses. Khichari and milk are recommended. Intake of coffee and tea should be reduced. Alcohol and cigarettes only aggravate the negative conditions.
8. *Fasting*: This is an excellent way of combating indigestion and quickly demonstrates to the sufferer that eating habits are the source of the problem. The habit of fasting for one day a week is highly recommended.

Further recommendations

- Try to develop self-awareness while eating food. This is a fundamental yogic practice. Be regular with meal times and strictly avoid eating between meals. Eat slowly and masticate the food thoroughly without being under any pressure to finish the meal. Try to extract maximum pleasure from each morsel of food, rather than unconsciously overeating.
- Always try to have the right nostril (pingala nadi) flowing when taking meals. This will increase the digestive fire.

- Never take food when you are anxious, excited or tense. Proper digestion demands that total awareness be focused on eating, and that the body and mind are relaxed. If the mind remains tense or preoccupied, the necessary digestive energies cannot be awakened and indigestion will result. If one is anxious or tense when food is being served, it is better to relax for 10 minutes in shavasana before commencing the meal.
- Avoid eating late at night as indigestion and disturbed dreams will result during sleep. A light evening meal should be taken around sunset and, if desired, warm milk can be taken before sleeping.

Peptic Ulcer

Peptic ulcer is a corrosive sore occurring at the lower end of the oesophagus, in the stomach wall, or in the upper part of the duodenum, just beyond the pyloric valve. Peptic ulceration is the end result of repeated bouts of gastric irritation, and sufferers usually have some prior history of indigestion and gastric disorders.

Many symptoms of ulcer are identical to those of the less severe upper digestive disorders, and as a result, it is frequently difficult to make the diagnosis of peptic ulcer upon symptoms alone. The definitive diagnosis of ulcer is usually made by barium contrast X-rays, where a clearly defined ulcer crater, filled with opaque dye and thus appearing white, may appear in the gastric or duodenal wall. Doctors now use a fibre optic gastroscope, a tube passed via the mouth into the stomach, to actually see and thereby diagnose the ulcer without having to perform major abdominal surgery.

Medical science recognizes two distinct types of peptic ulcer, depending on the site at which they have developed.
- Gastric ulcer (in the wall of the stomach).
- Duodenal ulcer, with slightly different symptoms and patterns of incidence.

Gastric ulcer
The major symptoms of gastric ulcer are gnawing mid-sternal pain aggravated by food, tenderness at the pit of the

stomach, vomiting and haemorrhage (internal bleeding). There is usually an associated loss of appetite and weight. The condition develops after frequent or long-standing bouts of less severe gastric inflammation (gastritis). The pain and the condition are aggravated by a rich, spicy diet, alcohol and smoking, while temporary relief is obtained from milk, bland preparations and by fasting.

The patient is commonly a young to middle-aged person who is thin or underweight with a tense and anxious personality. Gastric ulcer frequently occurs in an individual with a highly competitive and compulsive personality, who lives with a high level of tension. This person has a very low tolerance of frustration and is unable to forget achievement-orientated anxieties even for a moment. Unfortunately, such people often aggravate their condition by indulging in excessive smoking and/or drinking in order to 'calm down and relax'. Both these habits are gastric irritants in their own right, and serve only to further irritate the ulcer.

Ulcer victims are worriers through and through. They are eaten up by obsessive anxieties, which may be projected onto anything, including success, failure, performance, projects, fidelity, illness, betrayal, etc. The object of worry will vary from person to person but the factor of unrelenting worry is common to everyone.

Duodenal ulcer
Duodenal ulcers occur in the wall of the first part of the small intestine into which the gastric contents are emptied via the pyloric valve. The pain associated with a duodenal ulcer is a deep central abdominal one, which is relieved, rather than aggravated, by food. For this reason, the sufferer usually has a tendency to overeat and is consequently overweight. He or she frequently wakes up early in the morning with pain. Temporary relief may be gained by drinking milk, which has a soothing effect on the lining of the stomach and duodenum.

The cause of ulcer

Medical science and yoga are in accordance in recognizing that peptic ulcer is a psychosomatic disease. Experiments have shown that the lining of the stomach is an extremely sensitive recorder of our emotional states. It has been observed to blanch when a fearful or threatening situation arises and to blush red when rage and anger are expressed. Physiologists now recognize that emotional tensions and psychic stress factors, including high levels of frustration, are relayed to the digestive organs and glands via the sympathetic (solar plexus) and parasympathetic (vagus) nerve pathways.

In an individual possessed with gnawing worries, fears and constant frustrations, a constant stream of nerve impulses from brain centres in the limbic area and hypothalamus enters the autonomic nerves to stimulate a constant gastric acid secretion and turning over of the stomach. This goes on night and day, irrespective of whether or not there is food present in the stomach. Simultaneously, the same mechanisms are constantly being activated by oral stimulation of the digestive tract by smoking, drinking, and/or eating rich foods or continually 'grazing'.

Frequent bouts of indigestion, inflammation and irritation of the gastric mucosa result. Sensations of pain and irritation arise as the corrosive action of the highly acidic gastric juice (containing hydrochloric acid and pepsin) irritates the inflamed surfaces. Scarring and hardening of the mucosa ultimately occur. As a result, the mucosal resistance of the gastric or duodenal walls gradually diminishes and acid begins to burn a hole through the protective surface and into the wall.

Just as a sore anywhere on the body surface will not heal while it is constantly being aggravated, moved, rubbed and irritated, so a peptic ulcer, once formed, fails to heal while it continues to be irritated by acid secretions and the muscular wall continues to churn upon itself.

The mechanism of ulcer pain

The characteristic gnawing pain of peptic ulcer is produced when the acidic secretions find entry into the ulcer pit, where they cause intense irritation to nerves lying bare and exposed in the ulcer floor, like live electric wires behind a wall panel.

The whole psychophysiological process of ulcer pain can be summed up by the expression 'what's eating you?', for sufferers are literally eating themselves up by transferring unresolved mental conflicts, emotional tensions and anxieties into addictions and poor eating habits.

Possible fatal complications

Two rare but potentially fatal complications of peptic ulcer are perforation and haemorrhage. Perforation occurs when the ulcer penetrates right through the wall, spilling gastric contents into the sterile abdominal cavity. Haemorrhage occurs where the ulcer exposes and penetrates a major blood vessel, causing an enormous amount of blood to be rapidly lost. Both these complications result in shock and are surgical emergencies, which may prove fatal if proper medical care is not initiated immediately.

Treatment of ulcer

The ulcer sufferer is thus in a messy situation from which it is difficult to gain the necessary objectivity to escape. Medical measures alone are usually enough to bring a temporary remission of symptoms and anxiety, but ulcers inevitably recur when the former occupation, habits and lifestyle are resumed. For this reason, many doctors recommend the surgical removal of persistent gastric ulcers. Ulcer surgery usually involves severance of the parasympathetic nerves to the digestive organs and removal of part of the stomach itself. Even then ulcers frequently recur.

Doctors who utilize yoga in their practice have found that a combination of conservative medical management and yogic practices is the most effective way in which an ulcer can heal. Crippling anxiety problems can be effectively resolved, addictions overcome and a more balanced lifestyle evolved, even in the midst of the pressure and demands of modern life. The addition of yogic practices to conventional medical management enables the ulcer sufferer to implement specific lifestyle alterations which prevent a recurrence of the ulcer and the prospect of major surgery.

The role of drugs

Medical management of ulcers is largely concerned with relieving symptoms. It includes the use of antacid preparations which neutralize gastric acids and other agents which coat the gastric mucosa or inhibit the churning of the stomach muscles. These can be safely discarded under yogic management when healing takes place and symptoms disappear.

Yoga can definitely help the ulcer sufferer. It will show the way to a more balanced, enjoyable lifestyle based on daily practice of asana, pranayama and relaxation, a sound simple diet, freedom from bad habits and the anxieties and tensions that create them. Disease appears when such a lifestyle is lost, and disappears when the vital pranic energy needed for regeneration and good health begins to increase.

Yogic management of ulcer

Complete rest and a change of environment is highly recommended as the first step in ulcer therapy. This will enable the sufferer to completely forget about the tension of work, relationships, etc. A minimum of one month is usually necessary, and an ashram environment is ideal.

Initially, the ulcer sufferer should take a complete rest, sleeping on inclination, walking as desired but without exertion, and should be totally freed from any former commitments or responsibilities. Enormous mental relief will be experienced almost immediately.

1. *Asana*: Simple relaxing asanas can be introduced after two weeks, when initial healing has occurred and pain has been relieved. These must be performed in a non-competitive, enjoyable way, with emphasis on

relaxation and awareness. Pawanmuktasana parts 1 and 2 should be practised daily for two weeks, followed by surya namaskara to capacity in the second two weeks. Shashankasana and shavasana are recommended.

2. *Pranayama*: Bhramari and nadi shodhana will induce relaxation, if practised daily and without any strain.

3. *Shatkarma*: Neti and laghoo shankhaprakshalana can be introduced after some time, but kunjal is contraindicated in all ulcer cases because of the risk of disturbing the healing ulcer. Any patient with a history of vomiting blood or passing blood with the stool should not be prescribed kunjal kriya unless under expert guidance.

4. *Relaxation*: Daily practice of yoga nidra, which induces a state of mental and emotional relaxation, is most important in the resolution of anxieties and inner conflicts.

5. *Karma yoga*: Performance of some simple task in a non-competitive environment, e.g. carpentry or gardening for a few hours, is an excellent prescription for a formerly tense desk worker. Karma yoga brings mental release, relaxation and the potential for creative expression.

6. *Diet*: Initially a diet consisting of milk and non-acidic fruit is highly recommended to promote healing. Alternatively, a light liquid diet of vegetable broth, khichari, milk and bland fruits is acceptable. At all costs, spicy and heavy foods, smoking and alcohol should be avoided.

Constipation

Constipation is a very common chronic disorder of the lower digestive system in which the elimination of solid wastes from the body becomes slow and inefficient. As a result, there is a build-up of digestive and metabolic wastes in the large intestine, which becomes flaccid as it loses its muscular tone. As the disorder continues to develop, rotting wastes are held in store for longer and longer periods, resulting in a build-up or backlog of the body's wastes throughout the body tissues. The body begins to be poisoned by the build-up of its own wastes, just as a city chokes and becomes paralyzed if the garbage it produces is not continually taken away for disposal. Good health, high vitality and freedom from disease demand that the wastes be expelled regularly and efficiently.

Who is constipated?

There is no precise definition of constipation. The concept of ideal bowel function varies in different countries, climates, cultures, diets and individuals. No set rules can be laid down, but a number of guidelines can be recognized. Constipation has become an accepted way of life for many people today. Because of poor community education about basic health laws, they are unknowingly tolerating a degree of constipation for months and years, and this is rendering their bodily systems toxic and their minds dull, listless and heavy.

Simultaneously, their vitality and resistance to infections and degenerative diseases becomes very low.

A number of factors have combined to place modern men and women in this predicament. These include:

- *Sedentary lifestyle*: Constipation most commonly occurs in those who sit at an office desk all day. This leads to muscular stiffness, joint inflexibility, circulatory stagnation and blockage of pranic energy flow in the body.

- *Lack of proper exercise*: Many people today are either too busy, lazy or preoccupied to enjoy even a few minutes walk or exercise in their daily routine. They become averse to it. As a result, their muscles become weak and flabby, circulation becomes slow and irregular, and digestive and eliminative functions slowly deteriorate.

- *Poor dietary habits*: The quality of whatever enters the body via the mouth surely plays a decisive role in the quantity of the wastes expelled from the other end of the digestive tract. A diet which contains insufficient bulk or fibre, in the form of whole grains, fruit and fresh vegetables, inevitably leads to the infrequent and difficult passage of small, hard stools. The bowel works optimally when it has a large mass to contract against and propel along towards the anus, and such a bulk is provided by the fibrous cellulose residues of vegetables, fruit and whole, unrefined grains. In this respect it is the traditional poor man's diet which is most suitable for healthy bowel function.

The modern diet, based upon meat, eggs, oil, fats, cheese, milk and refined starch products such as bread and cakes, has little bulk but excessive protein, it takes a lot of energy to digest, and proves very constipating and heavy. In hot climates it proves particularly unacceptable. In colder, snowbound climates where it evolved, a heavier diet is required to maintain body temperature and insulation. Nevertheless, it necessitated the parallel consumption of alcohol as a mental stimulant, in order to overcome the resulting lethargic and heavy physical and mental state. It is a case where the detrimental effects of two individual poisons, when used concurrently, partly overcome one another. Many people on such a diet consider a bowel evacuation every two or three days to be normal, but this is too infrequent by yogic standards, especially when one considers that meat putrefies within twelve hours.

• *Toilet position*: The modern commode style toilet position for bowel evacuation is not the optimal one. It contributes to constipation by inhibiting the full relaxation of the lower colon and pelvic muscles. The best toilet position is the natural crouching or squatting pose, which allows full expression of the expulsive apana, providing more complete bowel evacuation.

Holistic medical approach

As has been noted previously, many people are constipated due to inadequate intake of high fibre foods, insufficient fluids and low levels of exercise. However, there is a very common disorder, called the Irritable Bowel Syndrome (IBS), which does not respond to these measures. People who suffer from IBS inevitably have one or more of the following: a) a food intolerance, b) an imbalance or deficiency of healthy gut bacteria (called probiotics), or c) an insufficiency of digestive enzymes, most commonly found in people who are protein depleted.

An appropriate investigation by a holistic physician or a competent naturopath will look for food antibodies of the IgG group and perform an assessment of gut function called Complete Digestive Stool Analysis (CDSA), which should provide the necessary metabolic information.

Mental constipation

Constipation is not only a physical condition, it is also a state of mind. A person whose thinking and lifestyle are uninspired, listless and non-creative is a frequent sufferer from sluggish digestion and constipation. Similarly, fixed

105

ideas and inflexible opinions, stubbornness and the inability to accept change gracefully often characterize the individual who accepts constipation as a fact of life.

'Constipation neurosis', or preoccupation with and fear of constipation, often occurs in individuals who have a great mental fear of letting go and accepting life's unpredictability and the certainty of change. Once the transitory, ever changing nature of our relationships and experiences is accepted, the bowels release their burden readily.

Students and people of intellectual temperament and occupation often complain of chronic constipation and bowel sluggishness. This is only natural as they dwell so much in their minds, usually at the expense of physical activity. The resulting imbalance between manas shakti (mental energy) and prana shakti (vitality) leads to their predicament. If some time is devoted in the morning to a simple asana program, and an evening walk is incorporated into the daily routine, the problem is often eliminated.

Yogic management of constipation
Even the most difficult and long-standing cases of constipation will be relieved by practising yoga techniques and taking a sensible diet and plenty of fluids.
1. *Surya namaskara*: Practise up to 12 rounds each morning at sunrise.
2. *Asana*: Pawanmuktasana part 2, kawa chalasana (crow walking), trikonasana, all forward and backward bending asanas, the vajrasana series of asanas (especially shashankasana), halasana, tadasana and tiryak tadasana, kati chakrasana, tiryaka bhujangasana, udarakarshanasana, matsyasana, ardha matsyendrasana, mayurasana. Sit in vajrasana for 10 minutes after each meal.
   In cases of mild constipation, drink one or two glasses of warm water before practising these asanas.
3. *Pranayama*: Bhastrika with kumbhaka and maha bandha, 5 rounds each morning. Surya bheda should also be practised, 10 rounds.

4. *Mudra and bandha*: Pashinee mudra, yoga mudra, ashwini mudra, uddiyana bandha, maha bandha.
5. *Shatkarma*: Agnisar kriya, nauli, basti and moola shodhana. Laghoo shankhaprakshalana should be practised each morning for up to 10 days, then twice weekly. Shankhaprakshalana should only be done under expert guidance.
6. *Meditation*: Antar mouna.
7. *Diet*: Eliminate starches from your daily diet and substitute fruits, vegetables, lots of salads and bean sprouts, whole grains and dried fruits such as figs and prunes. Prunes have an indigestible residue and thus provide bulk to exercise the intestinal muscles. Eat your food dry. If food is dry and then thoroughly saturated with saliva, it helps to lubricate the bowels. It will make the system alkaline and will greatly increase the rapidity of digestion. Drink plenty of fluids, including fresh juices which provide water in its purest form. Reduce the intake of salt.

Further recommendations

- The bowels should move at least once in twenty-four hours. On waking up visit the toilet until this habit of early morning evacuation is established.
- Moderate exercise after meals is very helpful. Never lie down or go to sleep immediately after eating, rather sit in vajrasana for a short while and then go for a short walk.
- Taking plenty of outdoor exercise, brisk walking, swimming, cycling and so forth, is essential for healthy digestion.
- Take cold baths only, both in the morning and evening.
- Laxative drugs should be avoided as they are very harmful and it is easy to form an addiction and become dependent on them for all bowel movements.
- After alleviation of constipation, adopt a routine of laghoo shankhaprakshalana and kunjal kriya once a week. Sunday morning may be the best time for these practices. Then let the next meal be mung khichari. This will prevent the recurrence of constipation.

Yogic management of haemorrhoids (piles)

This is a painful and troublesome condition in which one or more rectal veins become dilated and distended, prolapsing through the anal opening, especially at the time of defecation. This causes pain, bleeding and mucus discharge. The condition most commonly occurs as an effect of long-term bowel sluggishness and constipation, leading to excessive straining to pass the stools. As a result the drainage of blood from the anal area becomes stagnant and the veins become dilated and engorged with blood. Bleeding is precipitated by irritation when the hard stools are passed.

Natural history

Because of pain upon straining, the sufferer often avoids defecation, thus becoming even more constipated, and worsening the condition. After defecation, the piles can usually be manually replaced, at least in the earlier stages. Later on, this becomes increasingly difficult. Loss of blood is usually not severe, but may be sufficient to render the sufferer slightly anaemic, especially if it is chronic.

Surgical management

Haemorrhoids are commonly excised surgically by a variety of simple procedures, which give at least temporary relief from the condition.

Yogic therapy offers an effective alternative. Anyone suffering from piles and considering surgery is advised to apply yogic therapy for one month. During this period, many cases will disappear and surgery often proves unnecessary.

Yogic management

The first step in yogic management is to correct any underlying tendency to constipation. Without this fundamental restoration of normal function, little hope of relief from piles can be entertained.

Subsequently, a program of asanas, pranayamas and bandhas, followed by relaxation, should be adopted. The practices include moola shodhana (also known as Ganesh kriya), cleaning and massaging of the anus after defecation is completed. This should be performed by inserting the index finger well into the rectum and circulating it vigorously around the anal rim or margin. This stimulates the flow of prana to the region and promotes the drainage of pooled blood out of the haemorrhoids and back into general circulation. It should be performed up to 50 times in clockwise and anticlockwise directions, each time the rectum is emptied.

Yoga program for management of haemorrhoids

1. *Asana*: Pawanmuktasana part 2, shakti bandhas series, bhujangasana, ardha shalabhasana, shalabhasana, paschimottanasana, sarvangasana, halasana, vajrasana, marjari-asana, shashankasana, supta vajrasana, padmasana, yoga mudra. Sit in vajrasana for 10 minutes after each meal.
2. *Pranayama*: Nadi shodhana pranayama with jalandhara and moola bandhas, antar and bahir kumbhaka.
3. *Moola shodhana*: Daily, 50 times.
4. *Ashwini mudra*: anal contraction and relaxation, 50 times.
5. *Shatkarma*: Agnisar kriya, shankhaprakshalana, laghoo shankhaprakshalana.
6. *Relaxation*: Yoga nidra in shavasana.

Colitis

Colitis is a general term indicating an inflammatory condition of the large bowel. In India, the term is often used to indicate the mucus and diarrhoea which occurs with chronic amoebic dysentery, while in the affluent countries it refers to the chronic, psychosomatic disease of ulcerative colitis.

Two broad categories of this condition are usually seen – specific and idiopathic. The specific type of colitis arises from infections or infiltrations, such as amoeba and tuberculosis, though the latter form is quite rare today, so that amoebic colitis (amoebic dysentery) forms the majority of cases. The idiopathic variety is that type which cannot be traced to a specific cause, and its two most common types are ulcerative colitis and irritable bowel syndrome, both of which have a heavy psychosomatic component.

Signs and symptoms
The main symptoms of colitis are diarrhoea (frequent loose or watery motions often accompanied by mucous discharge), abdominal pain, tenderness and foul odour. In more severe cases, passage of blood and pus are additional symptoms.

The natural history of the disease is one of alternating attack and remission which often extends back for many years. During acute attacks the patient loses weight and becomes weak and anaemic.

The cause of colitis

Recent studies have shown that stress and strain are the major contributory factors in causing and aggravating the disease. Environmental stress, personal stress and stress resulting from natural calamities are important initiating factors. For this reason, the psychosomatic component of the disease must be considered in undertaking its treatment. A mild, temporary form of colitis can be recognized in 'student's diarrhoea', which afflicts many anxious college students in the weeks before major examinations, often forcing them to take recourse to the use of mild tranquillizers to see them through this tense period.

Medical management

Medical science has as yet made little progress in understanding and isolating the cause of colitis, and present management of the condition remains unsatisfactory. The physician is far more able to control the disease than to cure it. The control of diarrhoea via antibiotics, intestinal disinfectants and drugs to slow down the intrinsic nervous activity of the bowel have been the chief medicines used so far in treatment.

It was hoped that the introduction of the corticosteroids would revolutionize the management of diseases such as ulcerative colitis; however, the side-effects of these drugs are often found to be more serious than the disease itself, while their ability to control the primary condition remains limited.

The surgical approach to severe ulcerative colitis is to remove part or all of the colon. When the rectum is also removed along with the colon, the construction of an alternative opening in the abdominal wall is necessary. These procedures cause permanent and severe restrictions in the patient's lifestyle and if they can be avoided by using yogic practices, then both doctor and patient would agree that yoga should first be attempted for at least six months, if the condition allows.

111

Restoration of digestive power

According to yogic science, colitis is a syndrome which develops when the digestive power, agni, becomes imbalanced. As a result, disease producing micro-organisms can grow and the chemical and muscular processes deteriorate. Poorly digested wastes accumulate in the intestine and are passed in the stools. These micro-organisms and wastes are responsible for the foul odour. Yogic management aims at enhancing the digestive power so that formation of the offensive undigested wastes will be reduced and good health will supervene.

Yogic management of colitis

This program is recommended for these suffering from dysentery, ulcerative colitis, mucous colitis, irritable colon syndrome and nervous diarrhoea. It can be adopted to capacity, after the acute phase subsides.

1. *Asana*: Commence with the pawanmuktasana series parts 1 and 2, then the shakti bandha series. Begin the vajrasana series of asanas, then slowly progress to bhujangasana, dhanurasana, shalabhasana, paschimottanasana, sarvangasana, halasana, matsyasana, chakrasana, ardha matsyendrasana, mayurasana, padmasana, shavasana, sirshasana.
2. *Pranayama*: Sheetali, sheetkari, nadi shodhana and ujjayi.
3. *Mudra and bandha*: Vipareeta karani mudra, pashinee mudra, yoga mudra, ashwini mudra, moola bandha.
4. *Shatkarma*: Laghoo shankhaprakshalana, kunjal and neti. Agnisar kriya but not for ulcerative colitis, and only when the healing process is well and truly under way.
5. *Relaxation*: Yoga nidra should be practised daily and abdominal breath awareness in shavasana can be done whenever there is insufficient time for yoga nidra.
6. *Meditation*: Antar mouna has a prominent role in therapy, enabling the patient to recognize and counteract the subconscious psychic factors which are playing such a major role in attacks of colitis.

112

Dietary recommendation

In treating ulcerative colitis, a special diet which provides rest for the ulcerated colon is required. During the period of yogic therapy, the digestive power builds up most rapidly if the normal digestive processes are minimally activated. This applies to all forms of colitis. This is provided for by restricting the intake of normal foods, salt and water. In their place take milk.

Milk is an ideal replacement for the normal diet, which should be discontinued during the therapy period. Milk is a complete food which supplies all essential dietary elements, while leaving minimal waste residue. In recovery from colitis, the colon should remain free from irritation and therefore milk is the ideal food as it leaves the ulcerated colonic wall to heal itself in peace.

Simple khichari (rice, mung dal and vegetables cooked together) or porridge, place minimal demands upon digestive energy and can be taken in conjunction with a milk diet, though milk should be taken one or two hours before or after these light and easily digested foods because it does not mix well with other foods, even in normal situations.

In cases of dysentery (amoebic colitis), take 250 grams of curd (yoghurt), two teaspoons of sugar and three glasses of cold water. Stir the mixture and then strain the liquid through a clean piece of cloth into a clean vessel. To the same mixture add two or three glasses of water and follow the same straining process. It should be taken as frequently as possible. No food or any other drink (including water) should be taken until the dysentery has finished. Then gradually adopt the daily yoga program outlined.

Acute Gastro-Enteritis

Acute gastro-enteritis is a common acute illness with symptoms of abdominal pain and cramps, fever, vomiting, diarrhoea and loss of appetite. It occurs frequently in children when they have eaten unsuitable foods, or more than they need. Similarly, in adults it is a sign of dietary indiscretion or food poisoning. This form of illness is not a disease and should not be interpreted as such. It is a sign that some dietary abuse has been committed and that the body is seeking to heal itself. It only asks to be given a rest, including a rest from food for as long as the symptoms last.

General treatment
General fevers and diarrhoea of this simple kind should not be suppressed by drug management, as this only serves to prevent the body's efforts to eliminate waste matter. Rather, the best way to help is to conserve energy by fasting as long as the fever continues. This will ensure that the elimination is effective and recovery occurs rapidly over one or two days.

However, if the fever continues without dropping, or if marked dehydration is occurring due to continuing severe diarrhoea, or if the patient seems to have taken a turn for the worse and appears to be getting sicker, then expert medical guidance should be sought. It may be that the patient has contracted a more serious infection. A patient with cholera or typhoid is easily recognized and differentiated; he appears to be very sick and seems to be getting worse. This is the time and place to call a doctor, whose powerful drugs, which have no proper place in simple cleansing diarrhoeas and temporary fevers, may well save a life now. The difference between the two states is a matter of experience and common sense.

Yogic management of gastro-enteritis

Fasting with total bed rest in a quiet place is the best way to cure a simple fever, while eating is a sure way to prolong it. Short bouts of fever coming periodically, especially during a change of season, or following a period of overeating or indiscretion, are truly nature's blessings. They compel rest and enable the body to quickly readjust. They should not cause alarm as they are not sickness and no treatment is needed except rest. They are to be enjoyed, because they are a sign that health is strong and vital resistance is high.

During the fast, pure or boiled water should be taken. In cases of continuing fever or diarrhoea, a watery preparation of sweetened boiled barley can be safely taken. This interferes minimally with the elimination process, while helping to bind the loose bowels. When the fever has passed, the fast can be broken with fruit or vegetable juices or thin vegetable soup, followed by light khichari.

In general, the hatha yoga shatkarmas are contra-indicated during states of fever and acute illness. It is better to allow the body to eliminate wastes and purify itself at its own rate. Neti, kunjal and shankhaprakshalana are useful in more chronic states of disease or degeneration, where the body's ability to mount an acute purifying reaction is reduced. Here the need is to slowly and gradually build up the depleted vitality levels so that the body will again be capable of mounting its own purifying crises and acute reactions. This process of rejuvenation from states of debility and chronic illness can be greatly accelerated by yoga practices including intelligent use of the cleansing shatkarmas.

Asanas such as matsya kridasana and shashankasana are useful in relieving stomach cramps and pain. The best posture in which to sleep is matsya kridasana. Yoga nidra or abdominal breath awareness should be practised daily. Anuloma viloma and japa provide an effective means of diverting the mind away from pain and discomfort.

Malabsorption States

Malabsorption states refer to long-term disturbances of the processes of absorption and assimilation by the small intestine. These include sprue, Whipples disease and coeliac disease. They are characterized by gradual loss of appetite, indigestion, nausea, vomiting and diarrhoea. Sufferers usually loses weight, finding normal foods distasteful or repulsive. Their digestive powers become progressively weaker, and at the same time they lose interest in food and often in life as a whole. Anaemia, physical weakness and mental lassitude are common characteristics.

Malabsorption syndromes have much in common with cases of chronic hepatitis, in which listlessness, mental depression, loss of energy and interest in life are prominent manifestations.

Holistic outlook at malabsoption

Malabsorption is the end-stage of a process whereby the digestive system becomes so inflamed and depleted that it can no longer perform its function. It is a disease which may take many years, or even decades to manifest fully. Quite often, in the early stages, the inability to absorb is subtle, with only some nutrients being affected and the patient may just feel not as energetic as before. If the cause of this problem is not assessed properly and methodically, the digestive function will continue to deteriorate till the

117

symptoms become so severe that the individual begins to visibly waste away.

A comprehensive nutritional assessment, including digestive function, food allergies, vitamin, mineral and enzyme deficiencies as well as a detailed evaluation of protein status, will lead to an amelioration and eventually resolution of the problem.

Yogic management of malabsorption states

This yoga program is devised to help those suffering from poor digestive power, loss of appetite, weight loss, unexplained anaemia and failure to thrive.

1. *Asana*: Start by perfecting the pawanmuktasana part 1 series, then part 2. These are specifically designed to restore strong digestive function. They will awaken energy and relieve weakness and listlessness.

   After two weeks, change your program to the shakti bandha and vajrasana series, including shashankasana, shashank bhujangasana, marjari-asana and parvatasana. These will remove energy blockages in the lower psychic centres and direct it towards the middle digestive organs where failure of assimilation is occurring.

   Commence surya namaskara, working up to 10 rounds. Follow with total relaxation in shavasana, developing awareness of the abdominal breath. During this practice, centre your awareness on the abdomen and create the sensation of a mighty power being developed there.

   Finally, adopt five major asanas which activate the digestive mechanism controlled by samana. These are paschimottanasana, halasana, chakrasana, ardha matsyendrasana and mayurasana. In the final poses, direct your awareness powerfully to the seat of digestive energy. After each meal, sit in vajrasana for 10 minutes concentrating your awareness on the digestive process. Try to consciously enhance it.

2. *Pranayama*: Nadi shodhana pranayama stage 1 should be practised, 5 rounds to start with. Try to equalize and balance the flow of breath in each nostril.

After two weeks, commence stage 2 (alternate nostril breathing), 15 rounds. Try to develop control of the breath, which should remain silent and subtle. Work towards establishing the ratio 1:2 for inhalation, exhalation. Continue for one month. Then commence stage 3 with antar kumbhak and jalandhara bandha. Aim for the ratio 1:4:2, but do not strain. Continue for one month. Finally, practise stage 4. With antar kumbhaka, practise jalandhara and moola bandhas, and with bahir kumbhaka, maha bandha. Aim for a ratio of 1:4:2:2. This is extremely powerful in awakening the digestive prana and great inner heat will be generated during the practice.

Bhastrika pranayama with antar and bahir kumbhaka should be perfected next. Centre your awareness on the rising and falling diaphragm and visualize it as a bellows, fanning the digestive fire. Practise up to 5 rounds of 50 breaths.

3. *Shatkarma*: Kunjal and neti should be practised daily for the first two weeks. Learn to efficiently perform vyaghra kriya, the expulsion of undigested food remaining in the stomach, two to three hours after eating.

4. *Relaxation*: Yoga nidra should be practised with awareness of the abdominal breath, counting 50 to 100 breaths. Follow with chest and nostril breath awareness each for 50 to 100 breaths.

5. *Meditation*: Antar mouna stage 3, conscious creation and visualization of thoughts and feelings, should be practised while deeply relaxed. Generate the internal experience you feel when foods are consumed and visualize your digestive processes working optimally. Try to overcome your negative feelings towards foods. Feel them being absorbed into your body and feel energy flowing throughout the body as you digest them. Try to consciously overcome this psychological blockage.

6. *Diet*: Do not become fussy about food. While eating, do not allow yourself to lose awareness of the sacredness of what you are doing, and try to consciously grasp and

maintain the sensation of hunger. Do not allow it to slip away. Focus your awareness on the food you are eating and be aware that it is the product of the earth. Eat it joyfully, as prasad, a gift of the Divine Mother.

Eat simple vegetarian food. Do not cultivate whims for fancy foods and spices. Appreciate the nutritive value rather than the transitory taste sensations.

7. *Fasting*: Sometimes when you experience great hunger, deny it and avoid eating until the next meal. This is a most powerful way of removing psychological blockages, which inhibit a healthy appetite.

Diabetes Mellitus

Diabetes mellitus is a disorder in the metabolism of sugar. In the diabetic, the primary problem is the defective utilization of sugar by the body. Dietary sugars and starch are broken down to glucose by the processes of digestion, and this glucose is the major fuel for the various processes, organs and cells of the body.

Glucose metabolism is under the control of the hormone insulin, which is secreted by the pancreas, a large gland behind the stomach. When this gland becomes stressed or exhausted, the hormone insulin becomes deficient in quantity or sensitivity and the blood sugar level becomes high and uncontrolled as a result. The symptoms of diabetes are due to excessive sugar in the blood.

Diabetes is a very common disease today, especially in our affluent communities. Its incidence has paralleled the rising affluence of our lifestyle.

The cause of diabetes

Yogic science recognizes two interrelated causes of diabetes. Firstly, long-term devitalization and sluggishness of the digestive processes due to dietary abuse, overeating, obesity and lack of exercise. High intake of a sugar and carbohydrate rich diet is especially implicated.

If a person takes a large amount of sugar, sweets or chocolates, etc., their pancreas is ready to respond by

121

pouring out a large amount of insulin to rapidly manage the rocketing blood sugar level without incident.

However, if such a sugar-rich diet is eaten every day, the pancreas is being called upon constantly to secrete enormous amounts of insulin, and sooner or later it begins to tire and become depleted. Insulin production in response to sugar stimulation becomes increasingly inadequate. As a result, the blood remains saturated with sugar for long periods of time. It is then only a matter of time before diabetes is diagnosed. This usually occurs when the patient attends the doctor for investigation of one of the symptoms of high blood sugar, for example, an excessive thirst or urination, a resistant skin or urinary infection, or failing eyesight.

The second causative factor is that diabetes is stress related. The stresses and frustrations of modern sedentary humans are largely manifest on the mental and emotional planes, unlike those of our ancestors who had to wage a physical battle for survival. Nevertheless, the adrenal glands are in a constant state of activation, spilling the 'stress hormone' adrenalin into the bloodstream. This is a potent stimulus to the body to mobilize glucose into the blood. In this way a constant heavy burden of worries and anxieties imposes a constant demand for insulin secretion which can ultimately precipitate diabetes, especially in conjunction with a diet rich in sugar.

Two types of diabetes
The less prevalent but more severe form of diabetes occurs in young people. This is juvenile onset diabetes where the capacity of the pancreas to produce insulin has been partially or even completely lost. This may be due to a genetic defect, or may follow a viral infection or a severe psychic, mental or emotional trauma. This form of diabetes tends to occur in thin, sensitive, intelligent people. The medical treatment consists of daily injections of replacement insulin.

The more common form is late onset diabetes, which develops gradually in middle-aged, stressed, overweight, underexercised persons, whose diet contains an excess of sugars, starches and fats. This long-term overloading of the digestive system, especially the pancreas, leads to progressive deterioration of the insulin secreting mechanism and desensitivity of the body tissues to insulin.

In this form of diabetes, insulin is released in insufficient quantities and too late. Because some insulin producing capacity remains, this form of diabetes can be initially controlled through dietary restrictions alone. When this becomes insufficient, oral hypoglycaemic drugs, which decrease the blood sugar level directly are prescribed. At some later stage, due either to diminishing control or increasing side effects, these drugs are abandoned and the patient is put on daily injections of insulin, which will almost certainly be needed for life. However, with a system of regenerative yogic practices, it is often possible to cure this form of diabetes.

The dangers of diabetes

Because insulin is required to push sugar from the bloodstream into body cells, insulin deficiency causes high blood sugar but low intracellular sugar. Though sugar is freely circulating in the blood, it is useless because it is not being put to use by the body's cells. Therefore, the cells may actually be starving. It is a case of "Water, water, everywhere, but not a drop to drink!" The muscle cells which form the walls of the blood vessels are particularly affected by sugar starvation, leading to a whole range of degenerative vascular changes, including heart disease, arteriosclerosis, hypertension and kidney failure. Secondary effects of poor circulation, which are frequently seen in poorly controlled diabetes, include skin infections, gangrene, retinal destruction leading to blindness, loss of sensory nerve functions in the extremities, and impotence.

A blood sugar level which drops below normal, hypoglycaemia, poses a further dangerous problem for the diabetic. This can occur for a variety of reasons, such as excess insulin injection, and is probably the most dangerous situation the diabetic faces. Because the brain is totally

123

dependent on a constant supply of glucose, brain cells immediately begin to die of starvation when this supply is cut off. Unconsciousness (diabetic coma) and even death, will result unless sugar is rapidly replaced. Furthermore, when blood sugar is unavailable, the body releases fats from the storage tissues as a source of fuel. In burning this fat to produce energy, a state of high acidity (metabolic acidosis) results, which severely disturbs the delicate acid/base balance of the body. This is another frequent cause of death in uncontrolled diabetes.

The role of insulin

Before the advent of insulin replacement therapy, the diagnosis of diabetes was equivalent to a death sentence; its victims rapidly wasted away and died from starvation. They drowned in a sea of sugar. Insulin has certainly saved or prolonged many lives in the past fifty years. However, in the intervening decades it has been recognized that insulin therapy has certain drawbacks, as well as the inconvenience of lifelong dependence on daily injections. In recent years, yogic science has been found to offer an effective alternative treatment in controlling diabetes, especially before complications set in.

Holistic management of diabetes

The first important principle is nutrition. Many diabetics are overweight. This often causes the body's tissues to become resistant to the effects of naturally secreted insulin. Evidence shows that a diet high in protein and low in carbohydrates assists in increasing muscle bulk (which increases insulin sensitivity) and thus helping to diminish the fat mass. These changes alone can eliminate diabetes in some sufferers. In addition, a number of nutrients assist in improving the process of sugar metabolism and prevention of damage to the eyes, the nervous system, the kidneys, and the cardiovascular system, which are inevitable in any diabetic patient. These include vitamin C, lipoic acid, magnesium, zinc, chromium picolinate, vitamin E, B complex and selenium.

The yogic alternative

While medical science claims diabetes is incurable, many studies have proven that it responds very well to yogic management. In clinical trials, newly diagnosed diabetics have reduced blood sugar to normal levels and insulin dependent diabetics have been able to either discontinue insulin usage completely or have been able to considerably reduce their insulin consumption. The newly diagnosed diabetic has excellent prospects of completely controlling and correcting his condition if he adopts yogic practices and lifestyle under guidance.

Yoga does not accept that a lifestyle based on excessive consumption of rich food, obesity and lack of exercise is a natural or desirable state. To simply prescribe insulin or other drugs to counteract the effects of an unhealthy lifestyle is a disease promoting rather than a health promoting practice. The yogic treatment of diabetes is directed at the underlying causes of the disease as well as to its symptoms. It is based on the internal readjustment of the whole organism through stimulation of the body's own regenerative processes.

The yoga practices are thought to act in two distinct ways to overcome diabetes. Firstly it seems that the cells of the Islets of Langerhans, the secretory portions of the pancreas which have been prematurely exhausted due to oversecretion of insulin, are rejuvenated. This would mean that insulin production is stimulated and that its release is better timed so as to be appropriate to the level of sugar in the blood. This occurs gradually as depleted levels of pranic energy in the mid-digestive tract are restored.

Secondly, yoga seems to bring about a more general resensitization of muscle and fat tissues to the body's own (endogenous) insulin. This is achieved specifically by the anti-rheumatic series of pawanmuktasana, which removes blockage of energy in the peripheral muscles and tissues, and by the anti-gastric series of pawanmuktasana part 1, which selectively activates and mobilizes the body's fatty adipose tissue stores. Surya namaskara is a powerful pranic generator which also helps to restore a balanced metabolism.

125

Rejuvenating the pancreas

Rejuvenation of sluggish pancreatic secretion patterns in the diabetic occurs gradually by the performance of specific asanas, pranayamas, shatkarmas and bandhas, including uddiyana and nauli. These probably act by increasing the diminished flow of blood to exhausted and atrophied glandular segments of the pancreas.

Performance of the hatha yoga shatkarmas of laghoo shankhaprakshalana and kunjal kriya on a daily basis greatly aids the process of pancreatic restoration by removing toxic wastes from the whole gastrointestinal tract, and by cleaning and irrigating associated ducts and glands.

Provision of physiological rest is the greatest of all medicines in recuperation from diseases of depletion and exhaustion in any bodily system. The pancreas is no exception and restriction of dietary starch and sugars enables the gland to rest and recuperate from past abuse. Restoration of normal insulin levels in the Islets of Langerhans gradually occurs. This is aided by gradual withdrawal of external insulin injections in cases where the body has become accustomed to them. It is hoped that withdrawal will further stimulate the regenerating Islets of Langerhans to produce insulin in increasing quantities, until near normal levels are restored. Simultaneously, continual excessive mobilization of insulin is halted by adoption of correct diet, regular meal times, no snacks and not overeating.

Yogic management of diabetes

Yogic management of diabetes is demanding and it is best undertaken while the patient is fully resident in a properly equipped yoga ashram. At least one month should be allowed for the initial period of training and treatment, so that the new attitudes and practices can be thoroughly integrated into the patient's lifestyle.

It is important that diabetics undertake yogic therapy in conjunction with qualified medical supervision. Laboratory facilities should be available, so that progress in therapy can be objectively measured by serial assessment of blood and urinary sugar levels. This is especially important in the period of training when blood sugar levels begin to drop. The gradual withdrawal of daily insulin can be a dangerous procedure, and in our opinion should not be attempted lightly, as the risks of precipitating the patient into ketoacidosis and hypoglycaemic coma are considerable. However, with the proper medical collaboration this objective can be safely achieved.

Simplified one month yoga program

The yoga sadhana and progress will vary for each individual. This program should not be considered absolute for all diabetics, but should serve as a general guideline from which programs can be devised according to individual needs and capacities. Here is a general program of practices for diabetes management, modifiable according to individual needs.

First week

1. *Asana*: Pawanmuktasana parts 1 and 2, vajrasana.
2. *Pranayama*: Bhramari and nadi shodhana stage 1.
3. *Shatkarma*: Neti.
4. *Relaxation*: Abdominal breathing in shavasana.

Second week

1. *Asana*: As for the first week plus shakti bandha series.
2. *Pranayama*: Nadi shodhana stage 2; bhastrika (20 breaths).
3. *Shatkarma*: Kunjal and neti.
4. *Relaxation*: Yoga nidra.
5. *Meditation*: Ajapa japa stage 1

Third week

1. *Surya namaskara*: Practise according to capacity.
2. *Asana*: Vajrasana series.
3. *Pranayama*: Nadi shodhana stage 3 with jalandhara and moola bandhas. Bhastrika (30 breaths), with antar kumbhaka and jalandhara bandha. Sheetali and sheetkari.

4. *Shatkarma*: Full shankhaprakshalana once. Laghoo shankhaprakshalana each subsequent day. Kunjal and neti.
5. *Relaxation*: Yoga nidra (full one hour practice).
6. *Meditation*: Ajapa japa stage 2.

Fourth week

1. *Surya namaskara*: Up to 12 rounds.
2. *Asana*: Practise sarvangasana, halasana, matsyasana, paschimottanasana, ardha matsyendrasana, mayurasana, bhujangasana, gomukhasana.
3. *Pranayama*: Nadi shodhana stage 4 with maha bandha. Bhastrika with antar and bahir kumbhaka and maha bandha. Sheetali and sheetkari.
4. *Shatkarma*: Laghoo shankhaprakshalana, kunjal and neti daily.
5. *Relaxation*: Yoga nidra and prana vidya.
6. *Meditation*: Ajapa japa stage 3.

Further recommendations

- *Diet*: A low carbohydrate, sugar free, natural vegetarian diet should be adopted from the outset of therapy. Avoid rice, potatoes and all sugar products. Minimal spices, oils and dairy products. Eat wholemeal chapatis, leafy and watery vegetables, lightly boiled or steamed, salads and fruit.
- *Exercise*: Daily walking is recommended.
- *Insulin*: Withdrawal should begin in a stepwise manner at some stage in the first two weeks when laboratory results show that yoga is effectively lowering blood sugar levels. Continue reduction under medical supervision according to serial tests.
- *Drugs*: Oral drugs should be reduced and then stopped once yoga therapy commences.
- *Time*: Yoga program and dietary restrictions should continue for at least six months, and longer to prevent recurrence.
- For further information see *Yogic Management of Asthma and Diabetes*, published by Yoga Publications Trust.

Hepatitis

Hepatitis means 'inflammation of the liver' and refers to the acute derangement of the liver's structure following overexposure to specific chemicals, drugs or poisons and also after certain viral infections. As a result, the liver's myriad processing, detoxifying and excretory functions are temporarily suspended, as millions of its liver cells break down and die.

However, the situation is not nearly as gloomy as it sounds, for the liver possesses a remarkable regenerative ability and almost all patients will make a full recovery from a bout of hepatitis within a few months.

Specific causes of hepatitis

The liver can cease to function for a number of reasons. The most common causes are viral infections, poisoning with alcohol, and overexposure to specific drugs or chemicals.

Medical science has differentiated two distinct types of viral hepatitis. The first, type A or *infectious hepatitis*, is believed to be spread by faecal-oral contamination and occurs in epidemics. It is associated with poor sanitation and personal hygiene and commonly occurs in schools and institutions.

The second viral infection, type B or *serum hepatitis* is relatively rare and is considered more serious. It spreads by direct inoculation of the virus with transfer of blood or blood products by injection or transfusion. It is characteristically seen in health workers who deal with blood products and in drug addicts.

Drug-induced hepatitis is commonly encountered, parallel- ing the increased use of drugs and chemicals in both industry and the home. Most foreign substances, including modern drugs which are injected or taken orally, end up in the liver, which has the task of detoxifying them and preparing them for elimination from the body. A wide variety of modern drugs have been found to precipitate clinical hepatitis when given in high doses to experimental animals. They include several types of tranquillizers, steroid agents, antirheumatic medications, oral contraceptives and antibiotics.

In many cases, hepatitis has no obvious immediate cause, but it may occur due to long-term overstrain upon the liver's purifying and detoxifying mechanisms by an unsuitable diet which produces excessive metabolic wastes. These dietary factors include alcohol, meat proteins, rich fatty foods, spicy and refined foods, chemical preservatives, synthetic agents and drugs.

Symptoms and signs of hepatitis

The initial symptoms of hepatitis are fairly non-specific. The patient loses appetite and suffers increasing weakness and malaise. After a few days these symptoms give way to marked nausea, a rising fever, pronounced body pains and headache. At this stage the patient feels very weak, dis- orientated and nauseous, and the urine usually turns a dark yellow-orange colour, while the faeces become pale, bulky and smelly, due to absence of bile. In addition, the liver often becomes enlarged and tender beneath the right rib margin. Finally, jaundice supervenes; at first the sclerae (whites) and the mucous membranes of the eyes, and later the whole skin surface, take on a yellowish pigmentation.

Jaundice is an indication that the body can no longer metabolize bile or that the liver is no longer capable of processing the waste products of blood cell destruction. As a result, the level of these highly pigmented wastes in the blood continues to rise until they spill over into the tissues, staining the whole body in the process. The skin usually becomes itchy as a result.

The process of recovery

Fortunately, the process of hepatitis is usually self-limiting. The acute phase of the disease usually lasts for two or three weeks, after which a period of six weeks or more is required to restore depleted energy levels. Possessing remarkable regenerative capacity, the liver rapidly rebuilds itself. The most important factor in making a complete recovery is that the liver should be completely protected from harmful toxins during the crucial period of cellular regeneration. Total rest is essential throughout this period.

In isolated cases, recovery of the liver is postponed or the acute disorder recurs. This can continue for months or years, with a state of chronic digestive weakness, physical tiredness and malaise, nausea and an aversion and distaste for life. This is known as fulminant or chronic active hepatitis.

Where no known hepatic poison is being taken either in the diet or as alcohol, the cause can usually be traced to a deep-seated emotional disturbance. Often sufferers feel incapable of living up to the expectations set for them in life and are unable to express negative emotions overtly. They are forced to suppress anger as they attempt to live up to the expectations of those to whom they are emotionally attached. They may cling to sickness as the best way of avoiding confrontation with a distasteful reality. In such cases, the most effective therapy for this 'jaundiced' view of life is meditation.

Opposing the liver's natural healing processes on a long-term basis ultimately leads to chronic liver failure, with death by self-poisoning the inevitable result. This occurs as body toxins and metabolic waste accumulate and fluid balance is increasingly disrupted. The medical solution is a liver transplant.

131

Yogic management of hepatitis – the initial treatment
Yoga has a limited role to play in the initial recovery from hepatitis. The fundamental prescription is total rest, while avoiding any activities, foods or drugs which will hinder the process of liver regeneration. The healing process should be supervised by a suitably qualified person. The only yoga practices which are recommended in the recovery period are japa and yoga nidra with abdominal breath awareness, which promotes relaxation and healing. Asana and pranayama are contraindicated for at least six weeks.

During the initial period of recovery, fasting should be undertaken for a few days. Citrus fruits or juices and ripe papaya should be taken to relieve the nausea which arises as highly alkaline fluid from the liver and pancreas pours into the duodenum. Astringent foods such as radish should be taken regularly. Meat, eggs, spices, oil, butter and ghee should be avoided for at least six weeks and should be taken only sparingly after that. Meat eating and heavy protein foods treble the work of the liver. Alcohol should be scrupulously avoided for at least six months to a year and, if possible, so should most therapeutic drugs. Vegetable soup, boiled or streamed vegetables and fruits are recommended during the first two weeks of treatment. Then starches and grains can be slowly incorporated into the diet.

After the recovery period
Physical activity should be resumed according to capacity. Light physical exercise with slight exposure to the sun to promote sweating is advised to facilitate elimination of toxic residues during recovery from hepatitis. For two weeks or more, pawanmuktasana part 1, followed by abdominal breath awareness in shavasana and gentle nadi shodhana pranayama should also be performed daily.

Yogic program after full recovery
1. *Surya namaskara*: 3 to 7 rounds should be practised at sunrise.

2. *Asana*: Paschimottanasana, vipareeta karani mudra and shashankasana are particularly recommended for optimal recovery of liver tissues. Other exercises having a direct influence on the abdomen such as ardha padma padmottanasana, yoga mudra, halasana, merudandasana and its variations should also be practised when the healing process is under way.
3. *Pranayama*: Bhastrika, surya bheda, nadi shodhana.
4. *Mudra and bandha*: Vipareeta karani mudra, pashinee mudra and yoga mudra. The liver can be steadily strengthened by daily practice of uddiyana bandha (or agnisar kriya) according to capacity, commencing with 3 rounds.
5. *Shatkarma*: Laghoo shankhaprakshalana should be done soon after recovery; kunjal kriya and vastra dhauti can be performed twice a week. They ensure strong digestive capacity, high resistance to disease and maintenance of digestive fire.
6. *Relaxation*: Yoga nidra.

Provided all precautions are observed, one eventually recovers from a bout of hepatitis stronger and more purified than before, and the newly generated liver is more capable of effectively purifying the blood stream. It is an example of an evolutionary disease and after recovery every effort should be made to preserve optimal digestion and cleanliness of the blood by following a sensible diet in conjunction with a yogic lifestyle.

The Problem of Obesity

Obesity means excessive body weight. This imposes unnecessary strain on the body's various physiological systems, especially the heart, circulatory, respiratory and eliminative systems, and predisposes the person to the development of many serious metabolic diseases, including diabetes, hypertension, heart disease and arthritis. In addition it leads to lowered vitality, mental dullness and depression.

The most common cause of obesity is overeating, pure and simple. The problem is not only too much food, but also that the wrong type of food is taken. A diet composed of excessive oil, spices, starches, sugars and refined products leads to excess weight, while a diet based on natural grains, fruit and vegetables leads one automatically towards correct body weight and optimal health.

Obesity typically occurs in two types of people. The first type is the competitive, passionate, acquisitive person who eats too much too quickly, using food as a channel to release pent-up mental energy, unfulfilled ambitions and desires. Here there is an excess of *rajo guna*, the activating principle in the personality. The second type is the housebound person who overeats out of boredom. Here there is an excess of *tamo guna*, the principle of inertia, where lethargy and dullness predominate. As people put on weight, they tend to become even less happy with themselves and their appearance, and thus eat still more. In general we can say that overeating is due to frustration, where unfulfilled creative energy becomes wrongly channelled into excessive desire for food.

All obese people suffer from glandular deficiency in that their endocrine glands cease to function correctly, leading to mental, emotional and hormonal imbalance. A small number of obese people, however, suffer from a primary glandular disturbance or imbalance, usually of the thyroid, adrenal or reproductive glands.

Treatment of obesity

Almost all people with obesity will return to a normal body weight and an inspired life if a daily yoga program is followed with determination. The problem is that the obese individual needs inspiration and willpower. He or she needs to lift themselves out of a rut of habits and patterns based wrongly in food, and redirect their energies into more healthy, creative outlets. Yoga practice provides an excellent means for achieving this goal.

The tense rajasic overeater benefits especially from yoga nidra. He or she habitually sits to eat with a tense, preoccupied mind, takes an enormous meal wolfishly without really relaxing, tasting and enjoying it at all. They should learn to relax for ten minutes in shavasana before each meal, dropping the mental preoccupations and relaxing the digestive and other bodily organs. In addition, an object of awareness while eating helps enormously. For example, one may follow a formula of filling the stomach one half with food, one quarter with water and one quarter empty, or one may fill the mind with the idea that with every piece of food placed into the mouth, one is feeding Agni, the deity of fire. "I am feeding Agni. This is the mouth of Agni." This transforms eating into a form of meditation and awareness, which automatically ensures a reduction in the amount of food consumed.

On the other hand the bored, tamasic overeater should be initiated into karma yoga, some mode of self-expression

135

which will get him or her out of the kitchen, out of the house, away from the constant temptation of food and into some more stimulating and useful activity. As other interests awaken, the obsession with food will fall away.

Holistic management of obesity

Here, one uses the same approach as when dealing with late onset diabetes mellitus. Please see the chapter 'Diabetes Mellitus'.

Yoga program

1. *Asana:* These are essential to remove blockages, liberate prana, revitalize the mind and activate the endocrine glands. Obese people should be encouraged to practise to their limit, but never to exhaustion. Let them practise with enjoyment, relaxation and awareness, and their problems will fall away. It is not necessary to try to sweat off excess pounds. This is not the way to lose weight. The obese person has poor stamina and willpower and will soon drop out of such a demanding and exhausting regime. Permanent loss of weight demands a total overhaul of the pranic energy structure of the body and mind.
Asanas build up vitality slowly but surely. They rebalance the nervous and endocrine pathways gradually and effortlessly. In yoga the slimming and rebalancing process occurs on an altogether different level from the gymnastics program aimed at sweating off a few kilograms, at best a temporary measure. Weight will surely reaccumulate quickly unless the psychic and pranic energies are rebalanced and glandular mechanisms readjusted. Best practices are pawanmuktasana and the shakti bandha series, followed by surya namaskara. Major asanas, especially useful in balancing the endocrine glands and spinal nerves, can be adopted after some months of daily practice of these simple ones.
2. *Pranayama:* Bhramari and nadi shodhana are especially useful in awakening diminished vitality. Excessive

pranayama, which stimulates appetite, should be avoided. Mild bhastrika helps speed up the metabolism and reduce fat.

3. *Shatkarma*: Kunjal and neti should be practised daily, and poorna shankhaprakshalana should be practised once under guidance in an ashram. Laghoo shankhaprakshalana should continue once or twice weekly. These practices will relieve a clogged up and devitalized digestive system, overtaxed bowels, depleted liver and pancreas. As a result, long forgotten mental and physical lightness, increased vital energy and clarity of mind are experienced.

4. *Relaxation*: Yoga nidra is essential each day. A negative sankalpa (resolve) should not be adopted, as this is suppressive and may lead to overeating on the rebound. A positive resolve, in a form such as, "My vitality is increasing daily" or "My creative energy is being liberated from food more and more each day" is a powerful means of overhauling a faulty, uninspired lifestyle.

5. *Diet*: Fasting is not recommended for obese people as it is extremely difficult to maintain a proper fasting program, free from the inevitable rebound reflex of overeating. Rather the daily diet should be made wholesome with simple food, regular meal times and no snacks in between. Sugar, sweets, oils, spices, milk and milk products, rich and refined foods which overtax the liver, digestion and heart, should be vastly reduced, in favour of whole grains, fruit and green vegetables.

Obesity education

The community needs to be educated on the importance of eating for hunger and physical need rather than for taste. The fashionable belief that a fat baby is a healthy one should be discarded, as this penalizes the child, leading to a weight problem in adolescence and later life. A child who lives in a house where frustrations and creative energy are wrongly channelled into overeating develops a similar samskara and carries it into later life.

Diversion of the creative impulse and energies into eating leads to physical, mental and emotional heaviness and dullness. People with creative genius are very active and seldom obese. They are usually consumed with their work, often forgetting to eat in the process. Daily practice of yoga under guidance goes a long way towards rectifying wrong eating habits and towards the proper expression of instincts and desires in creative, inspiring, healthy ways.

Joints and the Musculo-Skeletal System

Arthritis

Arthritis is inflammation of the synovial joints of the body and is one of the most common of all disabling diseases, afflicting an estimated one out of ten people, thirteen million in the USA alone. Arthritis is a crippling degenerative process which can result in irreversible destruction of the joint. The condition is characterized by pain, swelling, redness, heat and loss of function in one or more joints. Those most often affected are the large, weight-bearing joints (hips, knees and ankles) and the small joints responsible for repeated, finely articulated movement, such as the fingers.

In the science of yoga arthritis is not considered to be a disease in itself, but as one symptom of a widespread metabolic and pranic malfunction which begins early in a person's life.

Yoga offers a way to arrest this process. In fact, in the early stages, before irreversible damage to the joints has occurred, a complete reversal is often possible. In the later stages, yogic practices can reduce drug dependency, maximize remaining mobility and function in the joints, and make the life of the arthritic more tolerable and acceptable. Remarkable restorations of function and a vastly improved outlook on life have been obtained in severely crippled patients who have followed a daily yoga program with determination.

141

The physiology of arthritis

The normal synovial joint is a remarkable self-lubricating, living structure. The ends of the bones which form the joint are covered with a hard yet resilient tissue called cartilage and are bound together by ligaments which surround the space between the bones (joint cavity). The joint cavity is lined with a delicate synovial membrane which secretes synovial fluid to lubricate the joint.

The cells of the joint depend on a fairly tenuous blood supply for their vital requirements. If the circulation of prana in a joint is blocked or deficient over a long period of time, the supply of blood and lymphatic fluid becomes sluggish and the joint fluid grows stagnant. When this occurs, the waste products and poisons of cellular metabolism build up in the lubricating fluid of the joints, rather than being efficiently transported to the skin and kidneys for elimination from the body.

Acidic wastes and toxins accumulating in the joint fluid irritate the sensitive nerve fibres in the joint, causing pain and stiffness. If the circulation of prana in the joint remains blocked for a longer period, the structure of the joint itself begins to degenerate. The joint fluid begins to dry up, the soft cartilage lining corrodes and the bones themselves begin to accumulate excessive calcium, forming new bone growth which limits movement. As the process continues, the whole structure of the joint is destroyed, movement becomes impossible, pain and deformity arise and the sufferer eventually becomes crippled.

The forms of arthritis

Modern medical science has recognized several distinct forms of arthritis. From the yogic point of view these are different stages of the same basic blockage of prana rather than different diseases. The underlying process is the same, but variations in the rate of symptom development have led to a number of diagnostic tags being assigned to different sufferers of arthritis.

Acute arthritis: This transitory condition is well known to all. It is a common symptom of many illnesses and infections, such as colds, flu, fevers and diarrhoea, and occurs because the viral or bacterial toxins liberated into the bloodstream during the illness readily accumulate in the joint fluids. This symptom usually diminishes soon after the purifying process is completed or the infection is overcome.

Gout: This is a special form of acute arthritis which seems to be due to dietary self-poisoning. Gout is suffered by people whose intake of proteins, especially red meat, exceeds their capacity to metabolize them. Uric acid, a toxic by-product of the digestion of protein, is usually excreted in the urine, but in gout it accumulates in the joint fluid also. Eventually acid crystals form in the joints, just as excessive amounts of sugar crystallize in a water solution. Gout exemplifies the significant role of dietary self-poisoning in arthritis.

Rheumatoid arthritis: This severe, crippling and rapidly progressive form of joint degeneration often occurs in young and middle-aged people, and is becoming increasingly common. Though the cause remains unknown in the majority of cases, it is frequently triggered by a severe emotional shock, or may be precipitated following the sudden introduction of foreign substances into the circulation, perhaps from the administration of a powerful drug, or an acute infection. If these foreign substances accumulate in the joint spaces, the immune system sends white blood cells there to wage a violent inflammatory reaction against them. Offending substances can be eliminated fairly readily from those tissues which have a good blood supply, but in the joint spaces, which are more isolated from the general circulatory system, their removal becomes more difficult. The joint tissues themselves are not attacked, but they are the battleground upon which the war is waged. This fierce inflammatory reaction can completely destroy a major joint within a few months. A period of remission follows, but the disease frequently recurs in another joint, until finally the body is left crippled and deformed.

Osteoarthritis: This chronic degenerative arthritis is commonly seen in middle and old age, especially afflicting those who are overweight, have a heavy or toxic diet and have avoided exercise. Osteoarthritis frequently develops in a joint which suffered injury earlier in life, the injury causing pranic and structural derangement which was not fully corrected at the time. Osteoarthritis may also be associated with an excess of calcium in the body, either due to high dietary intake, or to imbalance of the parathyroid glands in the neck.

Factors leading to arthritis

A number of factors, including mental and emotional stress and faulty lifestyle and diet, are responsible for upsetting the balance of central controlling mechanisms in the brain and endocrine system, on which the ultimate health of the organism depends.

- *Diet*: Overeating and an excessively rich diet, especially one based upon meat, animal fat, heavy fried foods, highly refined and synthetic foods, and excessive milk, ghee, sugar and salt, play a large part in initiating and aggravating arthritis. Constipation aggravates the disease.
- *Exercise*: Lack of regular exercise causes the joints and ligaments to become stiff and inflexible. Habitually sitting in chairs and rarely sitting cross-legged causes stiffness of the legs, hips, spine and shoulders.
- *Mental factors*: Deep subconscious tensions, suppression of emotion, fear and hypersensitivity can lead to rigidity of the personality, which is then translated into physical tenseness, allergies, endocrine imbalance and so on. Psychic rigidity – stubbornness and fear of letting go, leads to physical rigidity in the form of arthritis, rheumatism, fibrositis and constipation. Individuals with arthritis may fail to express their deeper emotions and feelings, especially anger, adequately. They will say things like, "Don't worry about me; you go out and have fun." Yet all the while they suffer internally and this

internalization of feelings creates poisons which upset the total body metabolism.

Modern medical treatment

Modern medicine has not yet fully come to terms with the overall dimension of arthritis. It concentrates on the relief of arthritic pain, but fails to treat and correct its underlying causes. A wide spectrum of drugs are prescribed, beginning with aspirin derivatives, which act both as analgesics (pain-killers) and anti-inflammatory agents. Aspirin is effective, although tolerance develops and increasing doses are required. Prolonged use of aspirin in large doses can have damaging effects on the stomach, liver and kidneys, so the patient is graduated to the next stage in drug therapy. More powerful anti-inflammatory agents, such as indomethacin and phenylbutazone, are prescribed until a tolerance once again develops or harmful side effects again preclude continuation.

The next step is the corticosteroids, which are analogs of the hormones secreted by the adrenal cortex. These drugs have serious side effects. The patient's own adrenal glands begin to degenerate or atrophy and the body becomes fat. Diabetes and high blood pressure can occur, body hair grows profusely, and calcium is leached from the bones, rendering them more susceptible to fracture. The final step is the surgical removal of the afflicted joint and its replacement with an artificial one. These joints prove quite effective, often lasting for years. Then, a further replacement becomes necessary; however, the patient may now be at an age when the trauma of a major surgical procedure can barely be tolerated.

Holistic management of arthritis

Osteoarthritis can often be significantly improved with glucosamine and adequate quantities of fish oil and flaxseed oil, all of which have anti-inflammatory effects. It is also worth avoiding the nightshade foods such as potato, tomato, eggplant, chilli and capsicum, for a trial period, as these foods are known to aggravate the arthritic condition in some patients.

Rheumatoid arthritis is an autoimmune inflammatory disease. There is growing evidence that it may be a reaction to large protein molecules absorbed from incompletely digested foods. These molecules stimulate the gut immune system to produce antibodies, which, unfortunately, cross-react with our connective tissues and can cause inflammation in joints and muscles. Comprehensive assessment and management of digestive function, food intolerances, gut dysbiosis, essential fatty acids and antioxidants will often lead to a significant improvement or resolution of the condition.

Yogic approach

Yogic management of the arthritic process is all-embracing and effectively complements standard medical measures. However, yoga will never advocate drug management of symptoms in isolation, while neglecting to correct the underlying deficiencies of diet, exercise, lifestyle and so on.

All therapy should ideally be learned in an ashram setting, to benefit from its positive and supportive energies. This is especially important if the individual is exposed to negativity at home or work, or if the family is creating a dependent attitude in the sufferer, for example: "Oh the poor thing, he is suffering so much. You must rest, dear, let me do that for you." Karma yoga is as much a part of the sadhana of the arthritic individual as asana and pranayama. A well-rounded program of yogic therapy includes the following elements:

1. *Asana*: The major series of asanas for prevention and management of arthritic conditions is the anti-rheumatic group of pawanmuktasana, which puts the body through its full range of movements and fully relaxes and massages all the joints. Before commencing pawanmuktasana, the patient should soak the limbs in cold and/or warm salty water to encourage blood circulation. As the flexibility of the joints increases, other

asanas can be added; however, never strain or inflict pain. Major asanas include shashankasana, marjariasana, shashank bhujangasana and akarna dhanurasana. Vajrasana should be practised after meals if possible. Ultimately, surya namaskara should be adopted to capacity. Six to twelve rounds each morning should prove sufficient to prevent further arthritic degeneration throughout life.

2. *Shatkarma*: Poorna and laghoo shankhaprakshalana, kunjal and neti are very important in alleviating constipation and eliminating any metabolic acids and other wastes which accumulate in the joints, bloodstream and tissues. Arthritis will never be fully cured while constipation remains.

3. *Pranayama*: Including abdominal breathing, nadi shodhana and bhastrika bolster the digestive and eliminative capacities.

4. *Meditation*: Meditative practices release pent-up mental and emotional tensions. Antar mouna stage 2, where thoughts are observed, is especially useful in recognizing self-limiting and fixed attitudes and behaviour patterns. Then in stage 3 the sufferer should be encouraged to create mental scenes in which he or she is expressing deep-felt anger and aggression, thus releasing suppressed emotional conflicts which contribute to arthritic rigidity, while at the same time remaining a detached witness. Deep relaxation and meditation will develop a positive state of mind in the sufferer.

5. *Diet*: The following simple diet will reduce pain and allow the eliminative and regenerative processes to work at optimum efficiency. A strong, clean digestive system readily absorbs all necessary nutrients from the following diet:
Cooked light grains and cereals in the form of wholemeal bread, chapatis, rice, millet, barley, etc.
Boiled pulses (dal) especially the lighter types such as mung, are a sufficient source of protein.

147

Boiled or baked vegetables, especially greens but not onions.

Salads using green leafy vegetables, celery, tomato, beetroot, carrots, cucumber, sprouted pulses, seeds and so on.

Fruits (except bananas), both fresh and dried, and nuts in small quantities. Instead of sugar, a little honey can be taken. Reduce intake of milk and dairy products such as cheese and ghee. Avoid highly refined, processed and synthetic foods, including white flour (maida).

As a rule, only fruit and vegetables that are in season and grown locally should be selected. If absolutely necessary, small quantities of white meats, chicken and fish can be taken occasionally.

Meals should be eaten between 10 am and 12 noon and between 5 and 7 pm. The midday meal should be the largest one and the evening meal should be lighter. This ensures that food is in the stomach when the digestive energies are high and digestion is well underway by sleeping time.

Missing a meal or fasting one day per week will ease pain, especially during acute phases, and accelerates relief and recovery of health. Do not take snacks or eat between meals.

6. *Amaroli*: Drinking one to three glasses of fresh urine per day, massaging the joints with old or boiled urine, applying packs soaked in urine, can all have a place in arthritis therapy, especially in long-standing cases which have outlasted analgesic or steroid therapy.

7. *Rest*: During the acute, inflammatory stage, rest is essential. Subsequently, periods of activity must be alternated with periods of rest.

8. *Exercise*: It is very important to maintain a determined and positive attitude towards activity and exercise, even to the extent of pushing oneself, in order to maintain a maintain an active, self-sufficient lifestyle. Walking,

swimming, gardening and other gentle forms of exercise help to keep the muscles strong and the joints limber, and can be integrated into the daily routine in conjunction with simple asanas.

9. *Heat and massage*: Total immersion in a hot bath and the local application of moist or dry heat, especially in winter, relaxes the muscles and loosens painful contractions. Heat also reduces pain and inflammation, increases the metabolism, aids elimination of poisons, speeds up the production of natural lubricants, reduces swelling and aids in the reabsorption of undesirable calcium deposits, bone formations in and around stiff muscles, ligaments and joints. After heat therapy, general massage of the joints and limbs towards the heart invigorates and relaxes the sensory and motor nerves, promotes circulation and irrigation of blood and lymph, and has an overall, relaxing effect.

10. *Mental attitude*: Above all, the arthritic person who undergoes yogic therapy must strive for patience and positivity, and try not to be discouraged by the pain and discomfort which will have to be endured at the beginning. It is well worth the initial struggle in order to break down the vicious cycle of disease which causes arthritis. Yoga nidra is most beneficial here and should be mastered as a form of pain relief and mental transformation which reduces drug dependency and pain sensitivity. The strength of mind gained and the joy which is experienced when the disease process is controlled and reversed is something that all sufferers with arthritis can earnestly aim towards.

Cervical Spondylitis

Cervical spondylitis is the name given to long-term stiffening and degeneration affecting the spinal column in the neck. It is characterized by pain and muscular spasm in the back of the neck and shoulders. Tension headache is also commonly associated. The pain may radiate into the shoulders, arms and forearms and be accompanied by sensations of pins and needles or tingling in the same general area. Movement of the neck is restricted, and muscular weakness and even wasting of muscles in the arms, giddiness and ringing in the ears are not uncommon.

In some cases of spondylitis, signs of vertebral degeneration in the neck can be readily seen on X-rays. However, paradoxically, an X-ray of the neck of many sufferers appears normal and healthy with little or none of the classical visible signs of degeneration. Visible degeneration includes narrowing of the intervertebral disc space so that the area appears worn away and new dense bony projections, called osteophytes, are seen. The foramina or bony tunnels through which the blood vessels run become narrowed. These blood vessels supply not only the spinal cord, but also the rear portion of the brain including the cerebellum and medulla.

Bony constriction of these vertebral arteries will cause decreased blood flow to the brain and faintness and giddiness will result. Similarly, bony overgrowth may impinge on the delicate cervical nerve roots emerging on either side of the vertebral column in the neck. Aches and pains in the arms and back will result.

The cause

Osteoarthritis of the vertebral bones of the neck may be precipitated by a previous injury. The neck is the most delicate part of the spinal column and is also one of the most vulnerable. Even a jerk due to a moving vehicle stopping suddenly can cause such an injury in the neck.

Damage can also occur as a gradual degenerative process, due to wear and tear of the joints, bones, muscles and ligaments of the neck. Hence it is more common after middle-age and especially in middle-aged sedentary workers who sit with their heads held rigidly forward the whole day.

Medical management

Modern medicine mainly offers physiotherapy as a remedy for this malady, in addition to anti-inflammatory and analgesic (pain relieving) drugs. Intervertebral injections of corticosteroids into the painful areas often provide effective pain relief by damping down inflammation in the short-term, but many sufferers report that their overall state worsens after receiving a series of the injections, with the pain becoming ultimately worse.

Physiotherapy often provides effective temporary relief, but rarely cures the condition. It is administered in the form of short-wave diathermy, massage, cervical traction and the wearing of a cervical collar.

Yogic management

Yogasana prove both palliative and curative in spondylitis, especially in early and newly diagnosed cases, where minimal changes are detected in X-rays. Asanas act by reducing muscular tension and spasm and also by correcting posture. In addition, they restore pranic balance in the neck, leading to regeneration of damaged tissues and reversal of abnormal bone growth.

The following practice program is prescribed for sufferers of cervical spondylitis. It should be adopted slowly and carefully under skilled guidance, and then practised each morning.

1. *Asana*: Pawanmuktasana part 1, especially poorna titali asana (full butterfly), skandha chakra (shoulder socket rotation) and greeva sanchalana (neck movements). The neck rotation exercises should be performed carefully. Vajrasana, shashankasana, shashank bhujangasana, bhadrasana, shavasana, akarna dhanurasana, makarasana, marjari-asana and sarpasana can be performed. Later on, as the range of pain free movement increases, the following asana can be gradually adopted: padmasana, matsyasana, yoga mudra, supta vajrasana, saral dhanurasana, and ardha matsyendrasana. Sitting still in padmasana, or other meditative postures, with the spinal cord straight and the head slightly back, for increasing lengths of time is very helpful. Avoid all other asana, especially inverted asana, until marked improvement in the condition occurs.

2. *Pranayama*: Nadi shodhana stages 1 and 2.

3. *Meditation*: Kaya sthairyam is most effective in spinal diseases and deformities. The head should be held erect but with the slightest tilt backward, the spine upright and shoulders relaxed. An experienced yoga teacher will demonstrate the position.

4. *Relaxation*: Yoga nidra in shavasana. A neck support in the form of a soft pillow may be necessary.

5. *Shatkarma*: Neti kriya daily.

6. *Diet*: As for arthritis.

7. *Additional aid*: A cervical collar is often helpful.

Back Pain

Backache is one of the most common disorders today. Every year in the United States alone an estimated two million new members join the ranks of the multitude of sufferers from chronic back pain, while in the United Kingdom the syndrome is second only to bouts of respiratory disease (colds, flu, bronchitis, etc.) as the leading cause of lost working hours in trade and industry. It is estimated that between 50% and 60% of the population will suffer from an incident of acute or more long-term back pain at some stage during their life.

In spite of the magnitude of the problem, a simple effective cure for backache has proven to be elusive to modern medical science. For this reason, most doctors lack confidence in treating backache patients effectively, and therapy often becomes a long, drawn out and frustrating affair for the doctor and the patient alike. As a result, the attitude of the chronic back pain sufferer is commonly a fatalistic and resigned acceptance of this painful condition – "till death us do part."

However, our experience is that this resignation need not be the case, for yoga offers a simple, effective and permanent cure for this troublesome condition. We have found that many chronic back pain sufferers who have resigned themselves to a life of pain after diagnosis of incurable spinal degeneration or early osteoarthritis, can be liberated from their problem, and from later recurrences, a few days or weeks after adopting a simple daily yoga program. Furthermore, the small percentage of patients (perhaps 5%) who are actually found, upon X-ray examination, to be suffering from prolapse of an intervertebral disc, prove to be equally amenable to yoga therapy.

What causes backache?

This question is hotly debated in therapeutic circles. However, recent studies have shown that the majority of backaches are caused simply by muscular insufficiency and inadequate flexibility of muscles and tendons. This clearly contradicts the popular prevailing belief that a high percentage of backache is caused by slipped disc, arthritis and degenerative joint disease, or organic conditions such as bone cancer, Pagets' disease and rickets.

Research studies

In one study, conducted jointly by researchers from New York University and Columbia University, USA, a random sample of 5,000 consecutive patients presenting themselves to hospital casualty departments complaining of backache were followed up. It was shown that in 81% of the cases, the back pain was found to have no connection with herniated intervertebral disc, tumours or organic conditions of any kind. For over 4,000 of the patients investigated, back pain arose simply, yet agonizingly, from muscular strain and stiffness.

A similar study, again of 5,000 patients, conducted by Dr W.D. Friedman of the I.C.D. Rehabilitation and Research Centre, USA, obtained almost identical results, concluding that in four out of five patients, acute back pain occurs simply because functional demand upon the back muscles exceeds their capacity.

The failure to recognize this simple fact is probably the major reason why back pain is so poorly treated at the present time.

The mechanism of common backache

The most common site of backache is the lower back, followed by the neck and the region between the shoulder blades. This pain arises when the muscles surrounding and supporting the spinal column are held rigidly and uncomfortably contracted over a long period of time. This situation commonly arises from long hours in uncomfortable car seats and office chairs. When this goes on day after day, the muscles gradually go into a state of tight painful spasm which becomes semi-permanent, as fibroblasts infiltrate the troublesome region, laying down fibrous tissues. These fibrosed areas can be readily felt as deep hardened bands and nodules within the tender back muscles.

Chronic backache tends to be worse at the day's end and is relieved by massage, heat, relaxation and bed rest. It responds readily and permanently to a program of yoga asana and relaxation aimed at increasing the functional capacity of the weak muscles.

Acute backache

Acute backache is usually a variation upon this theme. This is back pain of sudden onset and agonizing severity, which renders the victim completely immobile and helpless. This pain can strike at any time, especially in those leading a sedentary lifestyle characterized by lack of exercise and overweight, both of which contribute to functional inadequacy of the back muscles. Acute back pain commonly arises after a trivial jolt or insignificant movement such as a cough or sneeze. Agonizing pain accompanies every subsequent back movement, to such an extent that movement becomes practically impossible.

This is by no means a rare occurrence, for statistics suggest that between 50 and 60 percent of the population will suffer just such an incident sometime in their life.

When one is in this predicament, the first thing to do is to get into bed as soon as possible. The muscles surrounding the injured area quickly go into spasm to provide a protective

155

immobilizing splint, preventing all further movement of the area. By immediately getting into bed the body demands are reduced and the muscles can safely relax a little.

In the acute situation, severe pain can be effectively relieved by aspirin. The bed should have a solid wooden supporting base beneath the mattress.

Application of heat to the affected area by fomentation or hot water bottle also brings relief. Stiffness can be avoided by gradually moving the position in bed from time to time. Alternatively, relief may be gained by applying a cold compress (ice blocks in a cloth are ideal) and some patients obtain best relief from alternating hot and cold compresses every few minutes. Gentle massage several times a day also facilitates recovery.

Ninety per cent of cases of acute back pain will fully recover with a week of bed rest, with vast relief after a day or two. The problem then becomes one of preventing recurrence and yoga proves of great benefit.

Yoga program to eliminate simple backache

These asana should be practised for 15 to 20 minutes each morning without fail, followed by 10 to 15 minutes in shavasana. This program is specifically designed to increase the functional efficiency of the various muscle groups responsible for back pain and should be learned under expert guidance. Reassess the state of your back and general health after one month.

1. *For lower back muscles*: ardha shalabhasana, shalabhasana, ushtrasana, makarasana, bhujangasana.
2. *For shoulders and upper back muscles*: dwikonasana, sarpasana, bhujangasana, marjari-asana, kandharasana.
3. *Relaxation in shavasana or advasana*: with visualization of tight, congested back muscles relaxing, letting go of tension and flushing the area with fresh blood. Pranic energy is visualized flowing into the back muscles in conjunction with the breath.

156

Dietary recommendations

Correction of back pain is facilitated when a light vegetarian diet is consumed and excess weight is removed. Correction of chronic constipation often brings spontaneous remission of back pain. In this respect the optimal diet consists of whole grains, chapatis or wholemeal bread, pulse, vegetables (steamed, boiled or salad), fruits, nuts and juices. Avoid excessive sugar, milk and dairy products, oil, meat and spices.

Slipped Disc and Sciatica

Slipped disc and sciatica are two painful, closely related conditions occurring most commonly in the lower (lumbar) region of the back, usually due to excessive straining while bending forward.

Anatomy

The human spinal column consists of thirty-three individual bones, termed vertebrae, stacked one on top of the other and supported by the thick and powerful spinal muscles. The spinal discs are cushion-like, fluid-filled pads lying in between each pair of vertebrae. These discs act as shock absorbers, preserving the brain, spinal cord and internal organs from jarring and damage as we walk. They are filled with a thick jelly-like fluid and are held in position by strong ligaments attached to the margins of the disc and to the bony vertebra.

Description of the condition

Slipped disc occurs where excessive strain is brought to bear upon the lower back region, causing one of these discs to rupture and tear. As a result the jelly-like disc fluid inside protrudes outward and may impinge on a nerve root. The most common sites of this painful and immobilizing injury are in the lower back at the L4–L5 or the L5–S1 discs. The injury most commonly occurs while bending forward with the knees straight to shift a weight from the floor or while shovelling or weeding in the garden. It can also occur simply when releasing the clutch pedal while driving a car.

This painful and immobilizing injury usually occurs when a person with weak spinal muscles and ligaments due to a sedentary lifestyle applies an excessive strain to the back. It seldom occurs in seasoned labourers or manual workers, but is frequently seen in sedentary workers who are unused to regular exercise.

The onset of slipped disc is usually sudden and immediate. Something is felt to 'go' or 'tear' in the lower back, followed by a sharp, well localized, low back pain which may be agonizing. The sufferer remains incapacitated, either unable to straighten up again or else unable to bend the back even slightly, as this gives rise to immediate, severe pain. He or she is usually brought to bed or for X-ray examination soon after. Over the next few hours the pain continues to worsen until it is constant and unremitting. This occurs as the ligaments and tissues around the injured, protruding disc become engorged with blood and tissue fluids. The protective covering of the spinal muscles rapidly goes into tight spasm to prevent further painful movement of the area, and the delicate pain fibres supplying the torn disc and its ligaments become increasingly irritated. The whole area becomes inflamed, swollen and very tender.

Sciatica refers to a sharp, lightning-like pain which shoots down the back of the leg. It occurs if the herniating material from a ruptured lumbar spinal disc impinges on the delicate nerve roots emerging from the lower three lumbar and first two sacral segments of the spinal column which converge to form the sciatica nerve.

The sciatic nerves run down the back of each leg, supplying the skin and muscles of the back of the thighs, calves and soles. This is why sciatic pain may be experienced in the buttocks, thigh or calf, even though the root of the problem lies in the lower back region. In response to this pain the muscles of the back of the leg go into tight spasm, especially if the sufferer continues to walk, because each step stretches and further irritates the injured nerve roots.

Long-term prognosis and complications

Many slipped disc and sciatica sufferers have a long history of recurring bouts of crippling incapacity stretching back for many years. The slightest sudden strain, twist or bending movement is often sufficient to initiate the whole injury process once again. As a result, they no longer enjoy a full, active life. They may easily become dependent on analgesic drugs for pain relief and are forced to frequently take time off from work or household duties in order to rest in bed.

Usually their employers, colleagues and even family members are initially sympathetic, but may later come to regard the problem as a psychological one, being unable to comprehend a life punctuated by continual incapacitating bouts of back pain.

Sufferers often develop personality disorders as well, becoming depressed, niggardly or irritable. They are often labelled as 'whiners' or 'complainers' and others avoid their company. Marital, family and social relationships commonly deteriorate as the problem continues to recur. Supportive belts worn beneath the clothing are usually prescribed, offering some relief from the physical problem but no prospect of cure. This is the unfortunate predicament of many long-term sufferers.

People who have suffered from a slipped disc for a long time frequently come to surgery for removal of the troublesome disc and permanent fusion of the intervertebral joint. This procedure, which renders the lower spine permanently stiff and straight, may nevertheless provide relief to individuals who have come to a point of physical and emotional exhaustion and psychic depletion after many years of suffering. It is an alternative which is far from ideal, but which often appears to be the only solution available. Fortunately yoga offers an effective, less painful and far simpler solution to this difficult predicament.

Initial recovery and management

Slipped disc, with or without accompanying sciatica, demands immediate immobilization on a hard bed. Absolute bed rest is necessary while the ruptured disc heals and inflammation subsides. In the first few days, relief from pain can be gained by applying alternating hot and cold packs over the tender, inflamed area. Aspirin and a muscle relaxant may also be prescribed.

It is important that the spine be kept immobilized as far as possible, as total rest is the quickest route to recovery. No attempt should be made to walk or leave the bed for any reason. The sufferer should rest in a quiet room with minimal disturbance until healing is completed. Meals should be brought to the bed and for toilet purposes a bedpan should be available. This regime allows healing to take place in ten to fourteen days. However, occasionally, months are required for a severe injury. Yoga speeds up recovery if practised correctly.

Yogic therapy

The basic yogic practices for slipped disc and sciatica are the backward bending asana which strengthen the posterior ligaments and muscles holding the disc in position and promote the flow of blood into the lower spinal region. Backward bending asana should be practised to capacity, gradually increasing the time of practice each day in order to restore spinal stability and regain a full range of back movement. In this way normal activities can be gradually readopted, while surgical intervention usually proves unnecessary. Recurrences are prevented by regular, ongoing practice. We recommend the following program:

1. *Asana*: In the acute stage of immobilizing pain, a prone (face down) posture on a hard bed should be adopted. Resting in makarasana for extended periods reduces strain upon the disc and emerging nerve roots, providing relief of pain and promoting healing. Sleeping in advasana and jyestikasana is recommended. Matsya

161

kridasana with the affected leg drawn up to the chest to relieve tension upon the damaged nerve roots will bring relief. These postures should be adopted for relief of pain in the acute situation, so that as much total, undisturbed rest as possible can be gained. As healing proceeds and pain diminishes, the first asana to be attempted is the simplified version of bhujangasana, known as the sphinx asana. Aim to relax all tension in the lower back. If pain develops, lower yourself into advasana. Practise this 5 times. Once the sphinx asana has been mastered, the following asana can be adopted gradually in this order: ardha shalabhasana, sarpasana, saral dhanurasana, bhujangasana, shalabhasana, vajrasana, ushtrasana, meru vakrasana, bhu namanasana. Ultimately the program should be practised fully each morning. Each asana should be practised a maximum of 5 times and should be followed by complete relaxation in advasana.

Note: Avoid all forward bending asana for at least six months as these can precipitate a recurrence of the original condition. After recovery is completed, they may be reintroduced carefully under guidance, beginning with shashankasana, marjari-asana, shashank bhujangasana and the shakti bandha series.

Throughout the recovery period, the cross-legged sitting postures should be avoided, especially if they cause pain through increasing tension on the nerve roots in the lower back region. Pranayama and meditation in vajrasana are recommended.

2. *Relaxation*: Each session should conclude with deep relaxation for 15 or 20 minutes in advasana. Later on, shavasana can be adopted, and the longer practice of yoga nidra can be introduced.

3. *Ajapa japa*: Movement of breath awareness in the spinal passage from mooladhara chakra in the tail bone up to ajna chakra at the top of the spinal column is beneficial and effective in all spinal disorders, particularly slipped

disc and sciatica. It can be practised in any position with the spine straight. In the beginning, advasana will be suitable, though shavasana is better and should be commenced when the supine position can be adopted comfortably. Ajapa japa can be practised as frequently and for as long as desired as it speeds healing and brings deep mental and physical relaxation. As recovery continues, the practice should continue in vajrasana, and ultimately in one of the classical cross-legged meditation postures.

4. *Dietary recommendations*: At the outset a light, semi-liquid diet should be adopted. Vegetable soup is ideal. Khichari (pulse boiled together with rice or wheat) is also recommended. This conserves vital energy, redirecting it towards the important healing process. It will also prevent constipation which often proves a major problem for bedridden patients. Constipation invariably worsens and aggravates painful back injuries and rheumatic conditions.

As the condition improves, rice, pulses, and vegetables can be added and also wholemeal bread. Heavy, constipating foods such as meat, cheese and oily preparations are contraindicated. Dairy products (eggs, milk, ghee, etc.) should be avoided as extra protein is not required during this recovery period.

Prevention

The incidence of both slipped disc and sciatic injuries will be greatly reduced when those following a sedentary lifestyle, unused to back exercise or strain, learn to practise a few yogic asana daily to preserve strength and flexibility of the spinal muscles, discs and ligaments. Avoiding excessive use of chairs and back rests which weaken back muscles and learning to lift a heavy weight from the floor correctly – that is, from the squatting position with knees bent, so as to protect the vulnerable lower back from excessive strain and injury – will also preserve a healthy back.

Urogenital System

The Urogenital System

According to yogic physiology, the urogenital system is governed by the water element and the pranic energy by which it operates is derived from the psychic centre known as swadhisthana chakra. This centre of awareness in the psychic body can be contacted through concentration on the sacrum, or tail bone, at the termination of the spinal column, just above the anus, or on the bony pubic arch, just above the urethra (urinary outlet) in the front of the body. In the scheme of human evolution, swadhisthana represents the stage of expression and fulfilment of subconscious desires through the medium of the instincts and senses.

Resistant and recurring infection of the urinary and genital systems, for example, may frequently occur following a stage of personal evolution when instinctive life devoted to the passions and their fulfilment has been a ruling and predominant influence in life. The reverse situation also predisposes the person to various disorders. There is a failure to recognize and accept the instinctive side of human nature, which is instead repressed and denied proper expression due to deep-seated impressions of fear, guilt or inadequacy. In either case the balance between manas shakti and prana shakti, which is responsible for good health throughout the body, is disrupted in this lower psychic centre. As a result, the operation of the various physical organs in this region is also disrupted.

In the urinary tract the organs responsible for the formation, collection, storage and excretion of urine from the body are disrupted and the common urinary disorders manifest themselves. Common urinary disorders include disturbances of the kidneys, which can become sluggish, or in an extreme case may stop functioning altogether. This can result in severe fluid and salt imbalance throughout the body. Faulty discharge of urine from the bladder, with pooling and stasis, can also occur enabling infection from outside of the body to gain a hold in the kidneys.

Infections, inflammations and other diseases are the visible manifestations of an underlying deficiency, blockage or disruptions in the flow of pranic and psychic energy in the *pranamaya kosha* (pranic body) and *manomaya kosha* (mental body) which form the more subtle components of our individual human personalities.

The urinary tract

The urinary and reproductive systems are closely interconnected and cannot really be considered in isolation, especially in the male body, where they share a common passageway (urethra) via the penis for both semen and urine. The urinary tract begins with the kidneys, two fist-sized organs lying in the loin regions, against the back wall of the abdominal cavity on either side of the spinal column. Each kidney is composed of millions of tiny filtering units called nephrons, which filter the bloodstream, removing excess salt and water from the body and extracting waste products of cellular metabolism, including urea, uric acid, ammonia, oxalic acid and creatinine.

From the nephrons, the urine passes into numerous collecting ducts within the kidney substance, where it is concentrated. These ducts collect together in the inner medullary region to form the ureters, one of which emerges from the apex of each kidney. These two ureters pass down into the pelvis where they enter the bladder, which rests on the pelvic floor.

The bladder is an expansile muscular bag into which urine is continually being emptied from above. It has the capacity to expand automatically as the volume of urine increases. When the volume reaches a critical level, the brain receives a sensory nervous impulse and relays this message into consciousness, so that we become aware of the need to empty our bladder. In the pranic body, this mechanism is mediated by the flow of prana in the vajra nadi, which links the urinary and reproductive systems to the brain.

The act of emptying the bladder is under voluntary nervous control (expect in extreme cases of bladder overload due to withholding of the reflex to urinate). Disturbances of this mechanism can occur when control over release of urine is partially lost either for psychological or psychogenic reasons. This is known as the *irritable bladder syndrome*.

The reproductive tract

In both sexes, the final urinary conducting pathway, which emerges from the base of the bladder, is known as the urethra. In the male body the base of the bladder is encircled by the prostate gland, which secretes a milky fluid. Entering the gland are two spermatic cords (the vas-deferens), one from each side, which conduct the testicular fluid containing active spermatozoa from the testes. Beyond the gland, both urine and semen are discharged from the body through a single common urethral pathway through the penis.

In the female there is structural separation between the urinary and genital tracts. The female urethra passes directly from the bladder to the outside and is separate from the vagina. It is much shorter than in the male and this anatomical difference partially explains why inflammation of the urinary tract is found to be more frequent and troublesome in women.

Vajroli mudra

Many disorders of the urogenital systems can be systematically overcome by the practice of vajroli mudra (for men) or sahajoli (for women). This involves contraction and drawing up of the whole urogenital apparatus, commencing with contraction of the muscular walls of the urethra, such as occurs when the urge to urinate is voluntarily resisted. This technique must be learned correctly, in conjunction with pranayama and bandhas (psychic energy locks).

In kundalini yoga and kriya yoga, vajroli mudra is gradually mastered, giving the practitioner a high level of control over instinctive life and enabling him to become established in a state of consciousness where the instinctive desires are recognized in their seed forms (vasanas) and their energy harnessed, liberated and utilized on a higher plane of experience.

Kidney Stones

Kidney stones occur due to metabolic and dietary imbalance in the body and reflect disturbances of the body's fluid and acid balance. Under different conditions, various substances precipitate out of the urine and form sludge, sediment, gravel or large stones. Sediments or even stones may pass in the urine, accompanied by severe pain and blood (hematuria).

Types of kidney stones
There are three most common forms of kidney stones:
1. *Oxalate stones* are likely to occur with persistently concentrated urine and some people assume that a diet including too much oxalic acid enriched foods is necessary for stone formation. Such foods are spinach, tomatoes, rhubarb, etc., but this is yet to be scientifically proven.
2. *Calcium or phosphate stones* are large and staghorn shaped. They may form rapidly under excessively alkaline conditions, or where there is a disturbance of calcium metabolism. This could occur due to imbalance of the parathyroid glands, excess of calcium food such as milk, or where calcium is being mobilized into the circulation from the bones of the skeleton.
3. *Uric acid and urate stones* may form due to acidic conditions, for example, where a diet too rich in protein sources such as meat, fish and eggs is being consumed.

Kidney pain

Ureteric colic is an excruciatingly severe form of pain which arises when a stone of relatively large diameter enters the narrow ureter and begins its passage down towards the bladder. This pain radiates from the loin into the groin and may occur in recurrent bouts of two or three hours, or a single bout may continue for twenty-four hours or more. It usually comes on acutely, causing the sufferer to draw up his knees and roll about in agony. It is frequently accompanied by vomiting, profuse sweating and a great desire to pass urine (strangury), though only small amounts are passed. This is a clear sign that the urinary tract is obstructed.

The acute bout of agonizing renal colic may require a morphine injection for immediate relief and surgery may be indicated in chronic cases where the presence of one or more large stones in the pelvis or the kidney is detected.

Causes of kidney stones

A number of factors combine to lead to kidney stone formation. They usually occur in the presence of some metabolic disorder and when the urine remains persistently highly concentrated. An unsuitable diet containing excessive meat proteins, acid forming foods such as refined flour and sugar products, too much tea and coffee, chemically preserved and treated foods, pungent and sour condiments and spices helps to precipitate stones. An unhealthy diet congests and overloads the liver, and what the liver cannot effectively detoxify and metabolize is passed on to the kidneys. There it may cause inflammation or gravel and stone formation. The kidneys pass as much as possible into the urine, which is usually foul smelling and highly irritating to the urinary bladder. The long-term effects of this may be inflammation, ulceration and tumour formation in the bladder.

Other factors contributing to kidney stone formation may include excessive salt or reduced water intake, leading to a highly concentrated urine and obstruction to urinary outflow, and chronic urinary tract infection, leading to stagnant urine. Lack of exercise, especially prolonged immobilization in a recumbent position during convalescence or recovery from injury, is another precipitating cause.

Yogic management of kidney stones

Kidney stone formation can be prevented and old stones and urinary sediments removed by adopting the following yogic management program and general recommendations. Those who have suffered a prior bout of mild or severe renal pain or have recurring bouts are advised to adopt this program in order to prevent further recurrences of the condition. Large stones, however, may prove to be a difficult therapeutic problem and if yoga fails to bring relief, surgery may have to be considered.

1. *Surya namaskara*: Up to six rounds.
2. *Asana*: Trikonasana, vajrasana, marjari-asana, vyaghrasana, supta vajrasana, ushtrasana, shashank bhujangasana, shalabhasana, ardha matsyendrasana, naukasana, ardha padma paschimottanasana, ardha padma halasana, chakrasana, merudandasana, hamsasana, mayurasana, koormasana, dwi pada sirasana, tadasana, tiryaka tadasana, kati chakrasana, udarakarshanasana.
3. *Pranayama*: Bhastrika with bandhas.
4. *Mudra and bandha*: Pashinee mudra and yoga mudra, moola bandha, vajroli mudra, uddiyana bandha.
5. *Shatkarma*: Agnisar kriya or nauli practised daily. Shankhaprakshalana in an ashram environment. Laghoo shankhaprakshalana once a week.
6. *Relaxation*: Yoga nidra and abdominal breath awareness.
7. *Meditation*: Ajapa japa, nada yoga.
8. *Diet*: A fresh wholesome natural diet is recommended. Fruit, juices and lightly cooked succulent vegetables are recommended to alkalinize the urine. Avoid or reduce the intake of meat, eggs, fish and milk products as they produce uric acids wastes in high concentration. Avoid acid forming foods and highly refined flour and sugar

products such as cakes, sweets, biscuits, etc. Restrict the intake of tomatoes and spinach, which are high in oxalic acid. Decrease the intake of salt. Try to drink at least four litres of water per day, especially in the summer months. It is claimed that pears can dissolve kidney stones if up to a dozen are consumed per day.

9. *Fasting*: In conjunction with increased water intake fasting is highly recommended in order to flush, cleanse and purify a sluggish urinary system.

Further recommendations

- A short walk each day is recommended, particularly after the evening meal.
- Try to get some outdoor exercise at least once or twice a week.
- Parsley tea is said to be very beneficial. Take a small glassful every three hours.

Prolapse

Prolapse is a common problem for women and men throughout the world, but few people are aware of the alternatives available to help correct it. Apart from surgical intervention there are various yogic techniques which are designed to reintegrate the pelvic structures and which often prove to be more beneficial in the long term than surgical intervention.

Quite simply, 'prolapse' is a term to describe the falling out of place of an internal organ or body part, and is used mainly for prolapse of pelvic organs. The rectum may collapse into or even beyond the external anal sphincter, causing lower back pain on defecation and irritation with some pain in the anal area. The uterus may drop from its original position into the vagina, or in severe cases, protrude externally. This is not painful as a rule, and only a dull ache in the lower back is experienced. This condition is associated with frequency or inability to control the flow of urine so it may be passed when you laugh or cough.

Sometimes organs move from their original position and impinge on other parts in the pelvic cavity. Normally the uterus is anteverted, facing forward, but it may turn backward and lie against the rectum in which case it has retroverted. This may be a congenital condition (something which one is born with) or it may develop later from strenuous lifting, etc. If a retroverted uterus impinges on the rectum, it produces the symptoms of constipation and an uncomfortable sensation when seated. In pregnancy it can lead to miscarriage.

The condition of cystocoele occurs when the bladder protrudes into the front wall of the vagina. Rectocoele is the protruding of the rectum into the back wall of the vagina. The symptom presented in rectocoele is constipation. In cystocoele it is frequent urination. Because the bladder can never be fully emptied, urine retention (known as stasis) also occurs giving rise to recurring bladder infections.

Causative factors

Though there is not a lot of pain associated with these conditions, continual discomfort is experienced which tends to make you very concerned about yourself. An understanding of your inner framework and what brings about these conditions is helpful in alleviating anxiety and enables you to confront the problem with common sense.

The pelvic contents collapse because weakened ligaments and muscles fail to hold the organs in their correct position. The ligaments are fibrous structures and resemble strong ropes. These are attached to the bony pelvic wall and form a network in the pelvic floor offering their support to organs and anchoring them in position.

The very central point of this ligamentous and muscular framework is the perineal body, a fibromuscular node lying approximately two inches (five cms) inside the body above the perineum (the area between the anus and vagina). From this node, eight important muscles and their ligaments arise, plus connecting fibres to the rectal and anal canal. If this becomes damaged, the function of the whole supporting system is affected, and the organs drop out of place. Gravity pulls and draws the organs downward and because of weakened impaired support they are unable to resist its force.

Weakening of ligaments and muscles occur during pregnancy and labour or may occur due to straining caused by constipation or frequent bouts of diarrhoea. At the time of

176

childbirth the downward energies maximize and a tremendous amount of stress and strain is brought to bear upon the floor of the pelvis. This is also true in cases of diarrhoea or constipation. So these muscles need to be strong to facilitate the tremendous strain that is brought to bear on them during these periods.

The root cause
In kundalini yoga it is taught that the seat or source of the body's life force or energy lies in mooladhara chakra, the root or support centre whose physical counterpart is the same perineal body as previously discussed.

This node is considered to be the trigger point for the life force or shakti which is not only the fuel for our physical body, emotions and feelings, but also for our spiritual aspirations. The pelvic area which centres around the perineal body is very sensitive to emotional upsets and conflicts which block or deplete us of energy, creative potential and physical health and vitality.

It is extremely important to keep the perineal area strong and active. You can begin to strengthen and rejuvenate it through specific yoga practices which will help you to integrate and balance the energies responsible for physical, emotional, mental and spiritual well-being, so that you again become a healthy, happy and whole person.

Yogic treatment
If you suffer from prolapse or its complications, here is a specific yogic treatment for these conditions. With regular practice of these asanas, mudras and bandhas you will find that your condition becomes more manageable and may even fully correct itself, but do not expect immediate or miraculous results.

In the yogic treatment of prolapse, progress is generally slow, especially if the structural damage is severe and a ligament has been badly torn. Even if surgery proves necessary, the yogic practices will help one to prepare for surgery and afterwards help convalescence and prevent recurrence. When the structural damage is less severe and the ligament is only stretched or slightly torn, you will find yogic therapy most beneficial. During the course of your practice you will also discover that emotional instability, lethargy and depression become problems of the past, and you will enjoy a more energetic and fulfilled life.

1. *Asana*: Pawanmuktasana part 2 and especially naukasana, vajrasana, shashankasana, marjari-asana, bhujangasana, shalabhasana, vipareeta karani mudra or sarvangasana, paschimottanasana and kandharasana.
2. *Pranayama*: Nadi shodhana, bhastrika and ujjayi.
3. *Mudra and bandha*: You may practise all of them or choose the one which is most relevant to your specific conditions: ashwini mudra, vajroli mudra, moola bandha and uddiyana bandha.

Further recommendations

• Throughout the day sit in utthanpadasana, with both legs stretched out straight in front of you, in preference to other sitting postures. This position pulls the pelvic organs upward.

• Avoid sitting in the squatting position as it strains the pelvic muscles and pushes the organs downward. Excessive use of the squatting position over a long period of time may bring on prolapse in ladies who are weak in the pelvic area.

Urinary Tract
Problems in Women

Urinary tract infections

Urinary tract infections are classified distinctly according to the exact focus of inflammation and infection. Inflammation of the urethral passage which empties urine from the bladder is termed *urethritis*; inflammation of the bladder is *cystitis*; and infection of the kidneys, ascending from the lower urinary tract is *pyelonephritis*. In general, the higher the inflammation lies in the urinary tract, the greater is the pranic depletion, and the more deep-seated the infection, the greater the damage and physiological disturbance to the body as a whole.

Bladder infection

Inflammation of the bladder frequently occurs in association with excessive acidity. This can be caused by a diet which is too rich in starch and sugar or by certain forms of mental tension. People who suffer from gout, rheumatism, piles, diabetes and extreme nervousness often develop this problem. One of the immediate causes of bladder infection may be exposure to cold after perspiring, or it could be caused by injury or a fall, or as a consequence of an infectious disease. Sexual life can also initiate or aggravate urinary tract infections.

Symptoms of bladder infection include burning pain in the region of the bladder, frequent urination and a desire to pass urine even when the bladder is empty. The urine is

179

often cloudy and acidic, may contain pus or blood, and in many cases constipation is also present.

Kidney infection

Those who harbour long-term resilient bladder infections, or who have proved susceptible to them in the past, risk seriously damaging their kidneys. Pyelonephritis, kidney infection, may result if the inflammatory process continues to ascend from the bladder up the ureters to gain a seat in the kidneys. This destructive process which affects the whole body occurs when pranic depletion is marked, thereby lowering resistance. Disturbances of the body's excretion mechanisms and salt and fluid imbalance result in serious illness.

Long-standing inflammation of the kidneys, as well as many other causes, such as obstruction of urinary outflow and the resultant back pressure, can produce severe and irreversible damage. The end result is the state of *chronic renal failure*, where the blood can no longer be purified of its waste products, and the whole body becomes poisoned by the build-up of its own metabolic, toxic by-products. Death is the usual and inevitable result due to auto-intoxication of the body in its own wastes, unless life can be prolonged either with the aid of an artificial kidney machine, which filters the patient's blood in the process known as 'dialysis', or by kidney transplant. These are end-stage procedures which are better avoided if at all possible.

The role of antibiotics

Antibiotic therapy is an effective means of temporarily reducing the troublesome symptoms of urinary tract infection. However, antibiotics usually fail to provide a permanent cure, and flare-ups in the condition occur frequently or sporadically so long as the underlying pranic deficiency remains uncorrected. In fact, repeated courses of antibiotics will further weaken the system in the long run. For this reason we recommend that antibiotics be used if necessary to initially combat the symptoms, but treatment should not stop there. A more extensive program of yogic practices which systematically restores the underlying depletion of pranic energy should then be undertaken. In this way, the most resistant and tenacious infections can be overcome, especially when yoga and antibiotics are combined, and further infections avoided by regular yoga practice alone.

Urinary disturbances in pregnancy

The pregnant woman must maintain a high degree of health if she and her baby are not to suffer from disease. In pregnancy she is predisposed to a number of major problems, and the life of her baby and herself can be seriously threatened. In terms of the urinary tract, urinary stasis, ascending infections, kidney disturbance and water and fluid imbalance throughout the body occur more easily when the rapidly growing uterus compresses the bladder, causing urinary emptying to be further compromised.

Pre-eclampsia (toxaemia of pregnancy) is a dangerous and potentially fatal disturbance of salt and water metabolism in the final months of pregnancy. The mother's blood pressure rises rapidly and this is the most frequent cause of sudden maternal and foetal death or miscarriage. Its management remains one of the most difficult therapeutic problems confronting obstetricians. The defect underlying eclampsia is a latent weakness in the mother's urinary system which is unmasked by the added stresses and demands imposed upon her metabolism by the pregnancy. Such disasters can usually be avoided by practising yoga under guidance during early pregnancy.

Stress incontinence

The involuntary leakage of urine from the bladder, incontinence, may prove to be a problem for many women, especially after multiple childbirths when the body has not been restored and strengthened correctly, and also in old age. In the process of delivery, the bladder and urethra are under stress and are stretched severely.

As a result, some degree of urinary continence is lost, which may not be fully regained in the months after childbirth when the pelvic organs remain slack and stretched. Urine is commonly lost while sneezing or coughing, or when the patient is unduly anxious. This is known as stress incontinence. Women who practise yogasanas after giving birth easily regain urinary control and pelvic function, far more effectively than women who make no conscious effort to promote healing and tightening of the displaced organs. They are also found to preserve more shapely figures, and the ravages caused by childbirth can be largely avoided.

However, women who are anxious to take up a yoga program to restore their pelvic organs and preserve their overall figure after childbirth are advised to avoid all asanas in the immediate post-delivery period, unless under expert guidance. This restriction should continue for forty days after delivery, so as to ensure that initial healing is complete and to minimize the risk of bleeding after delivery (post partum haemorrhage). Gentle pranayama and meditation can, of course, continue immediately after delivery.

Yogic management of female urinary tract disorders

Yogic management of urinary tract disorders aims to restore depleted energy in the urinary and reproductive systems. When this underlying deficiency is corrected, infections can no longer gain a foothold in the urinary passage, and the level of resistance and health of the whole body is bolstered.

1. *Surya namaskara*: Start with one round and gradually build up the number to twelve rounds each morning at sunrise.
2. *Asana*: Shakti bandhas, ardha padma paschimottanasana, shashank bhujangasana, bhujangasana, dhanurasana, dwi pada kandharasana, chakrasana, vyaghrasana, sarvangasana, halasana, ardha padma halasana, ushtrasana, ardha matsyendrasana, vatayanasana, siddha yoni asana.
3. *Pranayama*: Nadi shodhana and bhastrika in combination with internal kumbhaka, moola bandha and jalandhara bandha, and external kumbhaka with uddiyana bandha.

Practise from one to five rounds. Up to ten rounds of surya bheda should also be practised daily.

4. *Mudra and bandha*: Vipareeta karani mudra and pashinee mudra. Sahajoli and moola bandha, up to thirty times daily. Maha mudra and maha bheda mudra, three times each at first. Later the number of rounds can be increased.

5. *Shatkarma*: Neti and kunjal daily. Shankhaprakshalana should be done before commencing the yogic program, preferably in an ashram environment, then laghoo shankhaprakshalana can be performed once a week.

6. *Relaxation*: Yoga nidra, each afternoon and/or at night, just before sleep.

7. *Amaroli*: So that the urine will be bland and non-irritating, three to four litres of water should be taken daily.

8. *Diet*: A light, low protein diet, free of meat and all irritating and stimulating foods is highly recommended. Refined foods, sweets, and spices should be avoided. Alcohol and tobacco should not be taken, and in place of tea or coffee a small cupful of barley water or parsley or other herbal teas should be taken three times a day.

9. *Fasting*: One day per week, or missing the evening meal every few days, provides energy required to throw off tenacious infections. A longer fast will cleanse the whole system, and if it is followed by a fruit diet, this will speed up the healing process. Fruits are rich in alkaline salts and help to overcome acidity.

Further recommendations

- Those with a tendency towards bladder disturbance or a history of urinary inflammation are advised to drink plenty of water to continually irrigate the urinary passages.
- It is also recommended that they urinate soon after the sexual act, when introduction of contaminating agents into an already weakened system is most likely to occur.
- Fortunately, yoga provides a means of arresting the process of degeneration before end-stage renal failure develops and life is threatened.

Menstrual Disorders

The female reproductive system is more complex than its male counterpart and therefore it is not surprising that it is subject to more frequent disturbances. Unlike the male reproductive system, where the major reproductive organs and glands are visible externally, the major organs and glands of the female system lie inside the pelvic cavity and are not visible, except for the breasts and vestibule or outer entrance to the vagina.

Disturbances of the menstrual and reproductive functions are extremely common and are a source of continual suffering for many women throughout their lives. In many countries the topic of reproductive function is traditionally veiled in secrecy and, as a result, many women do not fully understand the natural processes and cycles occurring in their bodies, or are misled by superstitions and false or inaccurate information. Many are too shy or ashamed to seek guidance and assistance when troublesome irregularities of function occur, while many others accept their problems philosophically or are not even aware that a disturbance is present and that a healthier state is possible.

Specific menstrual disorders

Amenorrhea or the absence of menstrual periods is normal in children and women after menopause, as well as during pregnancy. Menstruation also remains suspended for a variable time in women who are breast feeding their baby. Stress and worry, fear and anxiety, change of environment and diet can also be implicated. Hormonal deficiency and certain tumours must be ruled out by medical examination before yogic therapy is embarked upon.

There are two basic types of amenorrhoea:

1. *Primary amenorrhoea*: When a young girl does not menstruate, it is usually caused by poor diet and lack of fresh air, sunshine and proper exercise. Constipation and other symptoms of tension may also be present. When these causes are removed, menses usually appear. If the girl still has not begun to menstruate by the age of sixteen and a gynaecological and medical examination reveals no abnormality, there should be no cause for alarm. Sometimes absence or delayed onset of menstruation occurs in gifted or spiritually minded children, when there is strong pineal control over the pituitary gland. Artificial hormonal manipulation to induce ovulation and menstruation should be avoided unless it is proven that the child lacks the necessary hormones for full secondary sexual growth.

2. *Secondary amenorrhoea*: If menstruation ceases for a few months with no underlying organic reason, the recommended yoga program usually restores normal function.

Dysmenorrhoea and menorrhagia are the medical terms for problems of painful, irregular or excessively heavy menstruation. The underlying emotional and hormonal imbalance is readily rectified by a simple and regular yogic practice.

Disordered menstruation

Menstrual difficulty (dysmenorrhea) spawns as much wretchedness as the common cold and medical insight into this problem is equally limited. However, one researcher in this field, Dr Katherina Dalton (USA), has established that 'woman's pain' is not one, but two distinct problems.

Spasmodic dysmenorrhoea is characterized by cramps and acute pain in the lower abdomen with perhaps nausea or shakiness at the beginning of the period. It generally

185

appears in women under twenty-five and usually clears up when the first child is born.

Congestive dysmenorrhoea is associated with the terrible tension that doctors call the 'pre-menstrual syndrome'. A heavy, dull aching in the abdomen and lower back may begin up to three or four days before the bleeding itself. Some women notice swelling and tenderness in the breasts, swollen abdomen or a generally bloated feeling. Greater fluid retention may be reflected in a temporary weight increase of up to three kilos, and there may be some nausea. Headaches, general stiffness and constipation are common. The worst aspects are the irritability, depression and lethargy that make this time of the month so emotionally debilitating. Both the physical and psychic congestion lessen in intensity when bleeding begins and are relieved when blood flow is most profuse. This kind of menstrual problem is common to women of all ages from puberty to menopause and seems to get worse with every pregnancy.

Although medical science has not been able to detect beyond doubt the cause of this pain, Dr Dalton's evidence and that of Drs Carey and Pinkerton in Australia, indicate that both spasmodic and congestive dysmenorrhea are due to hormone imbalance. With spasmodic pain there is too much progesterone in the body, while congestive problems are due to an excess of oestrogen. Another researcher, Dr Elizabeth Connel, suggests that uterine cramps could be due to high levels of prostaglandin. This is a hormone-like substance produced by the lining of the uterus in great quantities just before it is shed. Lack of progesterone (i.e. too much oestrogen) also causes the body cells to retain sodium and lose potassium. This has severe consequences, for the transmission of impulses throughout the nervous system and brain depends on the correct sodium/potassium ratio. It seems then that hormonal imbalance is also the physiological root of emotional vulnerability during menses.

The symptoms of altering hormonal levels in the blood and the mental and emotional reactions to them build up to a crescendo in the days and hours preceding the onset of menstruation. Their severity varies from individual to individual depending on the state of her health and the ability to accept and flow with the cyclical, hormonally induced changes. A high level of pain and discomfort associated with the menstrual cycle often reflects a high level of physical and nervous tension in the body, and mental and emotional opposition to the process. This is why some women who are habitually tense and on edge tend to have difficulty with their menstrual cycles, while those who accept the process with calmness and poise, whose bodies are not run down or pranically depleted and whose nervous systems are relaxed, have no abnormal symptoms.

Doctors usually treat menstrual difficulties with pain relievers and hormonal supplements (birth control pills) and a certain percentage of women on oral contraceptives find their periods easier and the flow lighter. However, the pill is, at best, a risky business, most recently being linked to uterine cancers, and an increasing number of women prefer not to use it. Yoga, on the other hand, offers natural and effective methods without toxic side effects that extend far beyond the physical. It develops our awareness of menstruation as a useful part of our lives, rather than a curse, and offers the techniques to tame the hormonal cycle and use it for our spiritual evolution.

A period of heightened awareness
The monthly hormonal cycle of menstruation serves as a constant backdrop for the mental and emotional life of every woman, as well as being an important factor in her overall state of health. From the spiritual point of view, the days around the menstrual period are very powerful and auspicious for a woman to practise meditation and japa yoga. The period commencing three days before the onset and continuing for five days of menstrual bleeding and the first five days of the new cycle is a time when a woman gains a heightened level of awareness naturally, by virtue of the

187

altering hormonal balance. This is a time when her natural insight and intuition become very prominent, and it is a most powerful time for psychic awakening.

During this period sense perceptions, psychic receptivity and intuition spontaneously sharpen; for example, a woman may become very much more aware of smells, sounds, textures and tastes. She may feel unusual repulsions or attractions which really reflect her altered state of awareness.

Many women become frightened because of unusual perceptions and experiences and may mistake them for hallucinations or symptoms of sickness because they fail to understand what is actually happening. Much of the pain and suffering of menstruation is due to fear and tension. When yoga is used to rebalance the disordered muscular and hormonal imbalances which distort menstruation, and fears and tensions are relaxed, the process will be seen in a different light – as a blessing in disguise. It is a period in which access to a higher level of awareness is temporarily available and this should be met with confidence. Yoga and meditation are the means of transforming the menstrual period from a troublesome and unhappy experience into a natural doorway to the spiritual dimension of existence.

Any woman who is taking hormonal preparations to normalize her menstruation, or is facing hysterectomy, the surgical removal of the uterus, to relieve such symptoms, is advised to adopt the recommended daily yoga program for some months. By reducing tension and directing prana to the reproductive organs, restoration of proper functioning follows. Women who practise yoga regularly have found that period pain is eased almost immediately and completely eliminated within a few months. They are generally more relaxed and overall health and vitality are much increased.

Yogic management of menstrual disorders

Many women ask if it is safe to perform asanas during their periods. It is essential not to strain at any time, but apart from this usual precaution there is absolutely no reason to abandon your practices. One reporter comments: "A majority of doctors now believe that not only can women participate in any strenuous activity at any time, but that they actually benefit from it. A 1965 study comparing 65 women swimmers with 138 non-athletic students revealed that the swimmers had far less menstrual difficulty."

Sirshasana (headstand) and sarvangasana (shoulderstand) are not advised during menstruation, especially when it is disturbed. Vajrasana, shashankasana, marjari-asana, vyaghrasana and abdominal breathing in shavasana help to relieve cramp. Congestive period pain is relieved when the menstrual flow is at its peak and this flow is quickened by contractions of the uterus such as those in orgasm. This suggests that moola bandha could be particularly beneficial, although you must discontinue this practice at the very first suggestion of faintness or other unpleasant effects. Moola bandha should also be avoided in primary amenorrhoea, unless under expert medical and yogic guidance.

The following program should be followed throughout the monthly cycle. Unless there is profuse bleeding or debilitating pain, the practices can even be done during the menstrual cycle.

1. *Surya namaskara*: This will increase the pranic energy and balance nervous and endocrine functions. According to capacity, gradually build up to twelve rounds over a period of weeks or months.

2. *Asana*: The shakti bandha series is most effective in releasing blockages of energy in the pelvic region. Then siddha yoni asana, ushtrasana, marjari-asana, vyaghrasana, shashankasana, supta vajrasana, vajrasana, shashank bhujangasana, bhujangasana, shalabhasana, dhanurasana, sarvangasana, halasana, kandharasana, chakrasana, grivasana (particularly for late puberty and leucorrhoea), paschimottanasana, matsyasana, ardha matsyendrasana, utthanasana, pada hastasana, hanumanasana, sirshasana, tadasana. Inverted asanas are particularly recommended as they promote drainage of the reproductive organs and

189

enhance pituitary blood flow. They should be avoided only on days of heavy menstrual flow.

3. *Pranayama*: Nadi shodhana, ujjayi and bhramari are effective, especially in cases of headache, migraine and mental tension in general. Pranayama removes psychic tensions and mental irritability. In cases of cervicitis and prolapse, nadi shodhana stage 3, with moola and jaland-hara bandhas, proves most effective. Bhastrika enhances vitality and eliminates toxins and is recommended in cases of amenorrhoea and dysmenorrhoea.

4. *Mudra and bandha*: Vipareeta karani mudra, pashinee mudra and yoga mudra. Ashwini mudra, moola bandha and sahajoli generate vital energy in the reproductive organs. They will also stimulate the pelvic nerves and tone the sexual and eliminative organs. Maha mudra and maha bheda mudra are particularly recom-mended to alleviate premenstrual tension as they regulate the distribution of prana shakti in the body and induce physical, mental and emotional tranquillity. Those women who suffer from prolapse of the uterus should practise moola bandha and ashwini mudra in conjunction with the inverted asanas.

5. *Shatkarma*: Neti should be practised daily, and kunjal and laghoo shankhaprakshalana twice a week, as required. Remember, constipation greatly worsens pelvic con-gestion, pain and cramp and should be corrected as an important initial step in relieving menstrual disorders and leucorrhoea.

6. *Relaxation*: Yoga nidra is most important, especially in the days of mounting premenstrual tension prior to the onset of the menstrual period. It relieves mental tension, moodiness, depression and heaviness. If there is not enough time for the full practice of yoga nidra, relaxation in shavasana and concentration on abdominal breathing should be practised.

7. *Meditation*: Japa, ajapa japa, antar mouna, nada yoga or chidakasha dharana.

190

8. *Diet*: A wholesome vegetarian diet is the best for most modern women. Meat especially is found to increase menstrual pain, volume and duration. Fasting or taking a very light diet, free from spices, oils, meat and milk is particularly recommended in the days immediately preceding the period. Many women report that dietary changes alone have reduced the pain and heavy flow of their menstruation by more then fifty percent.

Further recommendations

- Plenty of fresh air and exercise balanced by adequate rest and relaxation is important in stabilizing and rebalancing the menstrual flow.
- A light, pure vegetarian diet emphasizing fruit, grains, lightly cooked or raw vegetables and iron enriched food should be taken prior to and during the menstrual flow. An alternative is to take only fruit for one day before menstruation and one or two days into the period. Avoid meat, coffee, stimulants, processed and artificial foods.
- The body and feet should be kept warm and not exposed to cold weather. Application of heat to the pelvic region relieves pain.

Leucorrhoea and
Vaginal Infections

The specifically feminine problem of leucorrhoea or excessive vaginal discharge is one which been neglected for far too long. From sheer lack of information and a sense of secrecy, many women become worried, ashamed and afraid of this essentially simple and manageable disorder. The same applies to many simple and easily treated infections. The underlying imbalance which causes leucorrhoea and chemical changes also allows infections to arise. Leucorrhea and infection can be seen as progressively worsening imbalances and loss of vitality in the lower pelvic region.

Natural vaginal secretions

Many women think they have leucorrhea when in fact they do not. It must be understood that a certain amount of vaginal secretion is normal and healthy. The walls of the vagina contain tiny glands whose specific function is continually to produce a cleansing and lubricating film of moisture. This secretion acts as protection for the sensitive tissues of the vagina, preventing them from drying, helping to wash out undesirable microbes. The vagina, like the eye, is self-cleansing. Just as the eye is bathed with moisture at every blink, so too is the vagina kept fresh by the constant flow of internal secretion.

Healthy vaginal discharge is usually transparent or slightly milky and may be a little slippery. However, the texture varies with the phases of the menstrual cycle. Sometimes it is thin and watery, at other times it is very white, and quite thick and sticky like jelly. The amount of secretion also varies from time to time and from woman to woman. It may become noticeable even in young girls several years before puberty. If the vagina is healthy, there is no smell and no irritation or redness of the vagina and surrounding area.

Leucorrhoea

Between the two poles of normal protective secretion and vaginal infection, lies a non-infectious, painless but excessive discharge called leucorrhoea. Leucorrhoea is normal vaginal secretion, only much more copious. It varies from woman to woman and what is normal for one person may be excessive for another.

While regular secretion may leave white or yellowish spots on your underwear, it usually dries quickly and does not cause discomfort. However, if your clothes are marked, if you feel constantly wet or have to change your underwear several times a day, then there is no doubt the discharge is excessive. Some women find it so heavy that they must wear sanitary napkins even between their periods. You might experience pain in the back, chafing of the thighs, or a 'full' feeling in the abdomen. These are similar to the early indicators of infection, but are less severe. Moreover, infection usually causes more frequent urination and leucorrhea makes it less. Leucorrhea is an abnormally profuse discharge, but a clean one and does not cause any itching or inflammation of the vagina or surrounding area.

Predisposing factors

Leucorrhea can be the first sign of cervical erosion (sores developing on the opening to the womb). This is usually seen in middle-aged women and it is estimated that about 95 percent of women develop such sores at some time during childbearing years, so it is well worth medical investigation. Generally doctors conduct a full pelvic examination and take a pap smear as the condition could be premalignant, that is, it may, though rarely, develop into cancer.

Most often though, leucorrhoea is just one signal from our bodies that we are generally run down and our resistance is low, due to lack of sleep, bad diet or nervous tension. Women who have diabetes or TB are particularly susceptible. The next most common cause of excessive discharge is hormonal imbalance. Women using birth control pills or IUDs (loop, copper, etc.) are especially prone. It may also become a problem just before or after menstruation, during pregnancy or menopause, because of the natural alteration of hormonal level at these times.

Diet is an important factor in leucorrhoea. Excess mucus from too much milk, white flour and polished rice is expelled in the form of bodily discharges, including those from the vagina. Highly spiced and fatty food, and large quantities of sugar also contribute to this problem. Diets high in processed sugar and refined carbohydrates also create ideal conditions for vaginal infections because they change the acidity level of the vagina and allow harmful bacteria to proliferate. Numerous women have reported that simply adjusting their diet has drastically reduced vaginal discharge. Leucorrhoea very often occurs in conjunction with constipation which is well-known to result not only from faulty diet but also from stress and tension.

Emotional factors are often unconscious and many women find it hard to admit to suppressing their feelings and their negative attitudes about their physical selves. This is particularly true in connection with the reproductive organs, which are still frequently considered unmentionable. Such unconscious doubts may be then expressed as leucorrhoea, the excess discharge being a symbolic attempt to purify ourselves.

Infectious diseases

Heavy vaginal secretion is a sign of imbalance and this creates an excessively moist condition that is ideal for the development of certain vaginal infections. The normal friendly bacteria that keep the vaginal environment healthy may be displaced when the natural balance is disrupted, allowing infections to develop. At the same time the female reproductive organs are very vulnerable to ascending infections because they lie closely exposed to the outside environment and are easily contaminated. *Vulvitis* (inflammation of the outer genital region), *vaginitis* (of vagina), *cervitcitis* (of cervix), *endometritis* (of uterine lining) and *salpingitis* (of the fallopian tubes) can smoulder on for months or years and may result in irreversible sterility.

In the case of infection, there is usually not only abnormal discharge, but also mild or severe itching, burning of the area around the vagina (vulva), irritation of the vagina itself and, occasionally, more frequent urination. The first signs of infection are lower back pain, cramps and swelling of the glands in the thighs and abdomen.

The main index of infection is the nature of the discharge itself. Irregular discharge is referred to as 'non-specific vaginitis'. The discharge may be white, yellow or streaked with blood. In some cases the walls of the vagina can be puffy with fluid or covered with a thick coat of pus. In certain infections, discharge may not be a problem.

Sexual activity is a common means of transmission of both urinary and reproductive tract infections from one individual to another. Excessive or unsatisfactory sexual activity is usually based in mental and emotional tension, boredom and frustration. It is self-centred, in that one partner seeks pleasure without thinking of the other's needs and wants. This depletes energy from the lower psychic centres, rendering both the genital and urinary tracts susceptible to infection via sexual transfer.

Venereal diseases such as gonorrhoea and syphilis are spread only by sexual contact and are also manifestations of this process. For this reason they cannot really be classed separately and distinctly from other infections of the urinary and reproductive tracts, which may or may not have been initiated by sexual interaction. These venereal diseases

195

are really in a separate category of yogic therapy which should not be confused with the treatment of other more common and less severe forms of infection. They are highly contagious diseases and will require a combination of both medical and yogic treatment; medical treatment always comes first in these cases.

The two most common sources of infection are monilia and trichomonas, both of which are normally present in the healthy body. With monilia or yeast infections, the discharge is thick and white and may look like cottage cheese or curd. It has a smell like baking bread and this negative association can make a woman feel sick at the mere smell of food. Monilia infections are also very itchy and irritate the whole vagina and vulva.

Trichomonas is present in the bodies of both men and women, and about fifty percent of women have this organism in their vaginas, but often without any discomfort. When the trichomonas population grows too large, it gives a thick foamy discharge that is yellowish-green or grey and is identified by an extremely unpleasant odour. It most often flares up after intercourse because of the irritation of the vagina, but it can also be passed on by wet towels, underwear or dirty toilet seats. When one sexual partner is found to have trichomonas infection, the other partner will also probably be a carrier, if not actually infected, and both require treatment.

Monilia and trichomonas infections are extremely common. It is a rare woman who does not pick up such an infection at least once in her lifetime. These disorders are in no way to be classed with such virulent diseases as syphilis or gonorrhoea, and there is absolutely no cause for shame or humiliation. The secrecy and superstition surrounding female sexuality has been known to prevent women from seeking help in the case of infection, and the effects have been disastrous. If treated early, vaginal disorders are a minor nuisance; if neglected, they become difficult to cure, lead to more complicated illnesses and can cause organic damage to the point of infertility. If ignored during pregnancy, the baby is also affected. Competent medical help backed up with preventive yogic practices will ensure relief and rapid recovery.

The fundamental rule in healing and regenerating any weakened system is to provide the optimal conditions for rest. Temporary abstention from sexual life is thus an important step in the yogic management of infections of the reproductive system, for it removes the constant stimulation and irritation which aggravate inflammatory disease. As physiological rest is given, coupled with a daily yoga practice program, both physical and mental relaxation occur and symptoms of pain, discomfort and inflammation diminish as healing is initiated. Once a certain degree of health is attained, sexual activity can be resumed and is usually found to be both healthier and more satisfying.

Holistic management of recurrent vaginal infections

One of the most common and irritating vaginal infections is caused by yeast, candida albicans, causing a condition commonly known as thrush. Antifungal creams can easily treat occasional episodes, but if the problem keeps on recurring, it suggests an underlying disturbance of the immune system and a high probability that there is a source of the fungus in the gut, which keeps reinfecting the vagina. A systematic assessment and management of nutritional adequacy and digestive function will go a long way to help remove this bug and at the same time support healthy immune function and improve resilience to future infections.

Restoring the balance

The most common cause of leucorrhoea and infections are generally low vitality and hormonal imbalance. For women the two are so intimately linked that they can be seen as simply two different ways of stating the same problem. Since this is the case, yogic practices can have decided benefits in relieving persistently excessive discharge. In the case of infections the

197

following practices should be incorporated with medical treatment, so that while medicines remove the symptoms, yoga removes the imbalance at the root of the disease.

1. *Asana*: Surya namaskara, vajrasana, shashankasana, marjari-asana, ushtrasana and shakti bandha series. Sarvangasana, vipareeta karani mudra, bhujangasana, shalabhasana, dhanurasana, chakrasana and paschimottanasana are for the more advanced practitioners.

2. *Pranayama*: Nadi shodhana, bhastrika and ujjayi further enhance vitality and balance the mind and emotions.

3. *Bandha*: the most relevant to leucorrhoea are moola bandha and uddiyana bandha.

4. *Meditation*: Yoga nidra and antar mouna short circuit the spiral of tension that disturbs hormonal balance and depletes prana shakti.

Further recommendations

- Strict personal hygiene is the first step in dealing with leucorrhoea. It not only prevents infections and minimizes discomfort, but also helps to put the mind at rest. Wash the anus and vulva regularly. Pat the vulva dry and try to keep it dry. Many vaginal infections are due to spilling organisms from the anus to the vagina, so always wash or wipe the anus from front to back. Use the traditional oriental squatting posture on toilet seats. It is not only more efficient but also more hygienic.

- Avoid nylon underwear, tights or pantyhose. Nylon retains both moisture and heat, providing a 'hothouse' environment that encourages harmful bacteria. Wear only loose-fitting cotton underwear or, when the discharge is not so heavy, none at all. Many undesirable organisms are killed simply by exposure to air, which also freshens and cools the vaginal area.

- Douching or washing the interior of the vagina can be an aid in preventing infection provided it is not overdone. The healthy vagina is rather acid, and this acidity acts as a barrier to infection. Since blood is alkaline, the acidity level drops during menstruation and women tend to be more prone to infection. At this time douching with a slightly acid solution will re-establish the normal pH and may have a preventive value.

Suitable solutions are one teaspoon of bicarbonate of soda to half a litre of warm water, or one teaspoon of vinegar to a litre of warm water. Coating the interior of the vagina and the vulva with curd (yoghurt) is also recommended by many women as an aid in curing infections. This treatment seems to be most effective when applied in the very early stages while the symptoms are quite mild.

• Sensitivity to and understanding of the signs of her body's functioning are the antidote to fear and an aid to every woman's confidence. Moreover, knowledge of the rhythms and the workings of a healthy body is the basis of early detection of any disturbance or disease whether physical or mental. This awareness is fostered by practising yoga.

Disorders of the Male Reproductive System

The male reproductive system is closely interrelated with the urinary system. The urethra is the conducting pathway from the testicles, prostate gland and bladder. It is shared by both systems as a common pathway for the secretory product of the reproductive glands called semen, which contains spermatozoa, and also for the excretion produced by the kidneys (urine).

The role of semen

The discharge of semen fulfils two important purposes in men. Each is distinct and should not be confused with the other. Firstly, emission of semen is necessary for the process of fertilization of the ovum to occur within the female reproductive tract, resulting in the production of a child. This is the reproductive function of semen. Secondly, and more importantly, seminal discharge is a means of releasing pent-up conscious and subconscious emotional tensions.

The release of semen for the purpose of producing progeny is a matter of choice, and is only occasionally and certainly not frequently required. However, the release of pent-up emotional tensions through the medium of semen is a regular, normal and obligatory event for most men. Ejaculation of semen occurs in the conscious state during the sexual act, and in the subconscious or sleep state in the form of nocturnal emissions, wet dreams or 'night pollution'.

How much is normal?

There are many misconceptions about what is excessive, normal, or deficient sexual functioning, and many men are very confused in this matter. Some believe that any seminal discharge whatsoever, whether in the waking or dreaming state, is abnormal and a great loss to the body. Others believe that sexual potency must be proved as often as possible, and abundant release of semen is healthy and commendable.

Both these views are extreme, reflecting the confusion which is the cause of many psychological problems, guilt complexes and neuroses in men the world over. It is true that excessive, uncontrolled and continuing loss of semen over a period of time is depleting to the vitality and weakens long-term health, but it is also true that feeling guilty about nocturnal emissions or suppressing the release of semen is a frequent source of mental, emotional and physical disease as well. The truth lies somewhere between these two extremes.

It is not possible to state precisely how frequently seminal discharge will occur in a man enjoying optimal health. This varies according to age, temperament, marital status, emotions, season, diet and so many others factors. However, the occurrence of two nocturnal emissions in a month, on average, can definitely be regarded as healthy for a normal man who is single and who does not practise masturbation.

The role of the emotions

The interrelationship between the emotional and sexual metabolism must be made clear. Our feelings, desires and fantasies originate in the mental plane, but their effects are closely mirrored in our bodily systems. The pituitary gland is stimulated to secrete interstitial cell-stimulating hormone (ICSH) into the blood in response to this inner emotional metabolism. This hormone in turn activates the twin processes of spermatogenesis and testosterone production in the testes, which enables the desires and feelings generated mentally to be physically expressed through the reproductive system. This response manifests as the release of semen.

Therefore, the demand for seminal release is initially generated in the mind and semen is produced as the end result. In this sense, semen is a waste product of the emotional metabolism, released via the ejaculatory reflex in much the same way that urea, a waste product of protein metabolism, is routinely released in the urine.

Spermatorrhea

If the emotions are excessively dominant or unruly, the production and release of semen will automatically be excessive, just as a heavy protein diet will result in urine with a high urea content. Therefore, spermatorrhoea or involuntary seminal discharge is a very natural process. Where wastes accumulate in the body without release, disease results and this is why periodic wet dreams are considered natural and normal for men and should generate no guilt or anxiety.

However, where the emotional metabolism remains wayward and uncontrolled for a long period, the resulting excessive seminal release can prove overtaxing on the body's metabolism, leading to diminished vitality, weakened health and development of degenerative disease during the later years of life.

Why excessive discharge of semen is harmful

In producing a continual high volume of seminal fluid, which contains an enormous force in molecular form, the bodily systems are heavily depleted of vital energy. The seminal fluid discharged in one emission contains an average of 400 million spermatozoa. When the turnover rate of shedding and discharge of the sperms is very rapid, the body must continually replace this loss using a constant supply of metabolic energy.

Each minute sperm is packed with an enormous amount of energy – enough to enable it to swim three thousand times its own length. In relative proportions, that is the same as the amount of energy used up by a six foot man swimming one and a half miles. That is the amount, proportionally, of our body's metabolic and vital energy, packed into each sperm cell discharged in a single seminal emission.

This energy is lost from the body, but where has it come from? It is derived from the nutrients of the diet, broken down in digestion, assimilated into the blood and constituted into the fatty protein structure of the spermatozoa. Metabolic energy is consumed every step of the way, especially in the metabolism of the quantities of dietary fats and proteins needed to continuously construct and energize a high turnover of spermatozoa. When semen is being constantly and recklessly discharged, its continual replacement demands that a diet rich in fat and protein be consumed. This diet consumes a far higher amount of energy in its digestion, assimilation and metabolism than a light, low fat and low protein diet does and thus imposes a higher working burden on the digestive organs and glands such as the liver and pancreas, on the heart, circulatory, transporting and eliminative systems.

As a result, the cells and tissues of the various organs demand replacement more rapidly, and the higher overall cellular turnover leads to greater expenditure of metabolic energy, accelerates the metabolic rate and permanently elevates the resting or basal body temperature. According to gerontologists, who investigate the ageing and degenerative process, elevation and acceleration of these factors, are the major causes of rapid physical degeneration, decay and early death of the human body.

Can seminal release be controlled?

If it is clear that semen is produced as the aftermath of earlier emotional metabolism which activated the pituitary release of ICSH, then we must also accept that production and discharge of semen is the normal and inevitable accompaniment of our inner emotional expression. Human emotions must be expressed and their products must have an outlet if physical and mental health is to be preserved. However, if a man has an emotional nature and experiences frequent seminal emissions, what can he do to preserve his health and vitality and reduce the loss of semen?

The question is not so much one of preventing the release of semen but of controlling its formation. When the formation of semen is controlled, the necessity for its release diminishes and vitality is gradually conserved. This is achieved by gradually controlling the emotional metabolism. A man who has a problem of spermatorrhoea, or excessive seminal discharge, has primarily an emotional problem, not a physical one. Control of the emotional tendencies of the mind is achieved through the practice of yoga, including asanas, pranayama and meditation.

The influence of yoga practices

Yoga is tremendously effective, both in harmonizing and balancing the nervous and endocrine systems, and also in developing awareness of the different mental and emotional states and fluctuations. Out of this awareness, stability and control develop in time. This is why a man who suffers from uncontrolled passions, excessive emotional expression and spermatorrhea gains great benefit by adopting a daily yoga program to develop mental emotional balance, so that the resulting pituitary secretions are reduced and the formation of spermatozoa and testosterone becomes manageable.

This is the only way to eliminate the problem of excessive seminal discharge because it gets to the root of the problem. Many men who try to suppress the release of semen without understanding its dependence on the emotional states are putting the cart before the horse. Yoga is a great boon to them for it relieves their problem and also eliminates their guilt and anxiety about the whole subject.

Towards a balanced emotional expression

The average man committed to marriage or some form of external emotional life should not practise yoga with an aim to stop seminal discharge, unless both partners agree. That would only create an unnatural situation, which would in turn create tension and disease and is unfair to the partner. Rather, he should use yoga to find balance and tread the path between the extremes of total suppression and excessive expression. For the average man, emotional expression is a fact and necessity of life. It is one of the fundamental bases of human relationship, family, social and community life.

The secret of spiritual life for men today is to live with a spiritual awareness while participating in worldly life. What is required is controlled expression, which develops with the practice of yoga on a daily basis.

Mastery of the serpent power

Complete transcendence of the influence and effects of the emotions is a state of spiritual realization attained by yogis. They do not kill their emotions, but by increasing absorption in the path of kundalini yoga, kriya yoga and dhyana yoga (meditation), they are able to transcend and refine the instincts and passions, so that the emotions are realized and expressed in a more universal way. In higher states of awareness, compassion (common passion) for humanity as a whole replaces attachment and passion for particular individuals. In the process, formation and release of semen diminishes, and the energy is redirected and absorbed in the spiritual quest as fuel for higher states of awareness. That is termed mastery over the 'serpent power' and leads to lower dietary requirments, decreased metabolic rate and rejuvenation and preservation of body tissues.

Yogic management of spermatorrhoea and excessive nocturnal emission

In the following program, internal purification of the bodily systems plays an essential role. The digestive, circulatory and eliminative mechanisms must be cleaned out and operating optimally if the metabolic processes are to be gradually slowed down and the whole process of mental, emotional, endocrine and reproductive waywardness is to be gradually harmonized and balanced.

205

1. *Surya namaskara*: Practise up to twelve rounds daily after taking a cold bath.
2. *Asana*: Begin with pawanmuktasana parts 1 and 2, vajrasana and siddhasana, and then perfect pawanmuktasana part 3, the shakti bandha series. After some months begin these major asanas: dynamic pada hastasana, bhujangasana, shalabhasana, paschimottanasana, sarvangasana, ardha padma halasana, ushtrasana, shashankasana, gomukhasana, eka pada sirasana, moola bandhasana, dwi pada kandharasana, matsyasana, ardha matsyendrasana, sirshasana, tadasana, pada angushthasana.
3. *Pranayama*: Bhastrika with inner retention, jalandhara and moola bandha, five rounds of fifty breaths. Sheetali or seetkari for a few minutes. Nadi shodhana stages 1 to 4 (with maha bandha). Perfect each stage for one month before moving to the next. Practise up to ten rounds.
4. *Mudra and bandha*: Vipareeta karani mudra and yoga mudra. Vajroli mudra and moola bandha should each be practised twenty-five times before meditation.
5. *Shatkarma*: Neti and kunjal each morning. Laghoo shankhaprakshalana daily for one week, then once a week. Full shankhaprakshalana should be practised in an ashram before commencing this sadhana program.
6. *Relaxation*: Yoga nidra should be practised before sleep, and whenever there is time for relaxation, practise abdominal breath awareness in shavasana.
7. *Meditation*: Practise either antar mouna stages 1 and 2 (learning to witness the mental and emotional reactions of the mind) or ajapa japa every evening.
8. *Amaroli*: Commence with one glass of the first midstream urine each morning.
9. *Diet*: Eat a light vegetarian diet with very little salt. Meat, eggs, alcohol, oily foods and all refined, chemically preserved foods should be avoided as they only serve to stimulate the passions. The intake of dairy foods should be reduced.

10. *Fasting*: One day per week of fasting or missing the evening meal proves very beneficial.

Further recommendations
- Take a cold bath or shower every morning and evening.
- Rise from the bed as soon as you wake in the morning and keep yourself constantly busy and occupied throughout the day.
- Learn to witness your internal emotional metabolism. When the mind becomes engrossed in sexual thoughts, try to remain a witness to its influence on the reproductive organs and glands.

Sterility and Impotence

Sterility and impotence are two disorders where there is failure of sexual and reproductive behaviour for either physiological, anatomical or psychological reasons. Approximately one third of all childless marriages are believed to be due to sterility or infertility on the part of the husband. Seminal analysis is a relatively simple procedure which will indicate a lowered sperm count in the spermatic fluid, as well as the presence of abnormal or immobile sperm forms. This chapter deals with sterility and impotence due to malfunction of the male reproductive tract.

Yogic practices prove most effective in restoring both fertility and potency in men who have psychological, physiological or mild hormonal imbalance. Frequently a low sperm count is only a temporary state, and lowered and abnormal sperm counts have been corrected to within the normal range within three to six months of persistent yogic therapy.

Sterility

Sterility, which refers to the state of infertility, occurs in several forms. Sometimes it is due to faults arising in the chromosomal mechanism of sex determination as early as conception. In other cases it may be due to later developmental errors in sexual differentiation of the embryo and foetus up to the time of birth, and after birth in the ongoing sexual development.

Our anatomical, psychological, personality and behaviour characteristics are influenced by hormones, particularly the levels of the androgenic (male) hormones such as testosterone. Underdevelopment of the reproductive organs is termed *hypogonadism*. It includes failure of production of spermatozoa and the secretion of hormones. The defect may involve only impaired spermatogenesis in the seminiferous tubules of the testes, or it may also involve the interstitial (Leydig) cells, causing reduced testosterone levels. Where testosterone levels are reduced, failure of spermatogenesis is one inevitable result. Another is the diminution of the secondary sexual characteristics.

Sterility may be due to failure of the hypothalamic or pituitary secretion mechanisms upon which the gonads depend. In other cases brain and pituitary are intact, but there has been injury or destruction of the testes themselves. This may occur due to an accident, tuberculosis, gonorrhoea, syphilis, malignant tumours or orchitis. Surgical castration is another cause of sterility. Mal descent, or failure of the testes to descend into the scrotum from the abdominal cavity during the last months of intrauterine life, also leads to failure of development.

Where an injury or defect is one-sided, leaving the other testis unaffected, sterility will not result, because sexual and reproductive behaviour can proceed normally with only one operational testis. Cases of sterility due to organic causes such as tuberculosis, tumour, venereal disease and surgical castration are often irreversible. However, the vast majority of infertile men do not suffer from any of these organic causes and the outlook for them is more promising.

Signs and symptoms

The results of deficient or absent testosterone production depend on the sufferer's age at the time of onset of the disease. When it occurs before puberty, the genital organs and the secondary sexual characteristics such as beard growth, deepening of voice, etc., fail to develop. The sufferer is often excessively tall because of the failure of the long bones to stop growing at puberty. The typical prepubescent sufferer develops into a tall, thin man with a hairless face, a high-pitched voice, small genital organs and an immature personality.

Where the onset of sterility and testosterone failure has occurred after puberty, the resulting changes are less striking. Growth is not affected and there is regression rather than disappearance of the secondary sexual characteristics. The external genital organs undergo partial atrophy. Usual complaints are of fatigue, loss of initiative and decrease of sexual desire (libido).

Holistic management of male infertility

One of the major signs of male infertility is either a low sperm count or poorly developed sperm which are incapable of fertilizing an ovum. To produce adequate numbers of healthy sperm, we need to minimize or (preferably) eliminate the use of recreational drugs, avoid pollution with heavy metals such as lead, mercury and cadmium, and avoid volatile organic compounds (especially petroleum derivatives). In our industrialized and globally polluted world, this can be quite difficult. However, there are some nutrients and antioxidants which help to counter the effect of these toxins. These include vitamin B 12 1 mg/day, vitamin C 1–2 gm/day, natural vitamin E 400 mg/day, essential fatty acids, zinc citrate 30 mg/day and organic selenium (called selenomethionine) 200 micrograms/day.

In addition, keep up the intake of a variety of fresh fruits and vegetables, which have a wide range of nutrients and antioxidants not necessarily found in some supplements.

Impotence

Impotence refers to the inability of the male to participate in sexual intercourse because of a lack of sexual power. In the majority of cases it is due to psychological causes rather than to any organic abnormality of the testes or sexual organs.

210

Sometimes impotency results from dislocation or misalignment of one of the sacral or coccygeal bones in the termination of the spinal column following a fall, injury or strain. Impotence is also one of the symptoms of diabetes. An aversion for sexual intercourse may stem from traumatic experiences in early life which have led to unconscious attitudes of fear, guilt shame or inadequacy. In these cases, the technique of relaxation in yoga nidra can remove the root problem.

Often there is an associated blockage of pranic circulation in the pelvis and the lower psychic centres, known as mooladhara and swadhisthana chakras, and in extreme cases nervous weakness or paralysis in the lower limbs may develop. These cases usually respond to regular meditation and yoga nidra, in conjunction with asanas which specifically tone and activate the reproductive organs. They should be practised on a daily basis. The shakti bandha and vajrasana series are highly recommended, as well as paschimottanasana and bhujangasana.

The practices of moola bandha, vajroli and ashwini mudra arouse dormant energy and overcome pranic, psychological and mental deficiencies and blockages.

Dietary experts suggest that impotence may be caused by a deficiency of vitamin E in the diet. Recommended foods include olive oil, wheatgerm, sesame seed, unfired cereals and peanut butter as well as milk and other dairy products.

Yogic management of sterility and impotence

It must be remembered that successful impregnation, fertilization and subsequent pregnancy always involves the cooperation and interaction of husband and wife as one. Frequently it is impossible to determine by laboratory tests where the defect lies in cases of infertility in marriage. Often husband and wife are each psychologically and physiologically normal. Yet some aspect or condition of their sexual interrelationship remains unfulfilled or unfavourable. For this reason, both partners are recommended to adopt a yoga program and practise it together.

1. *Surya namaskara*: Practise up to twelve rounds each morning at sunrise.
2. *Asana*: Begin by perfecting pawanmuktasana parts 1 and 2, then the shakti bandha series. After one or two months commence the following major asanas: vajrasana series, particularly shashank bhujangasana, marjari-asana, supta vajrasana, and ushtrasana.
   Then dynamic pada hastasana, bhujangasana, shalabhasana, paschimottanasana, sarvangasana, druta halasana, matsyasana, gomukhasana, dwi pada kandharasana, kandharasana, chakrasana, hanumanasana, bhadrasana.
3. *Pranayama*: Nadi shodhana and bhastrika with antar and bahir kumbhaka, jalandhara, uddiyana and moola bandha. Surya bheda should be practised at the time of sunset for ten rounds.
4. *Mudra and bandha*: Pashinee mudra and yoga mudra. Vajroli and moola bandha should each be practised thirty times a day.
5. *Shatkarma*: Neti daily and laghoo shankhaprakshalana whenever constipation is present.
6. *Relaxation*: Yoga nidra and abdominal breath awareness in shavasana.
7. *Meditation*: Ajapa japa while seated in siddhasana.
8. *Amaroli*: If the man drinks the urine of his wife daily for a minimum period of three months, as enjoined in the ancient tantric texts, this may aid a successful pregnancy. In many previously childless marriages, including those in which the cause was attributed to psychological impotence, lowered or abnormal sperm count and hormonal or endocrine deficiency developing after puberty, this technique has been a boon.
9. *Diet*: A high protein diet is recommended and all grades of meat may be included if desired. Milk and dairy products such as ghee and cheese are also recommended. This diet will accelerate the metabolic rate and provide the raw materials for increased spermatogenesis. However, constipation should be avoided by taking honey,

fruits and nuts. More vitamin E enriched foods should also be added to the diet. These include pure peanut butter, olive oil, wheat germ, sesame and unrefined cereals and grains.

Further recommendations

- Overwork, mental fatigue and physical exhaustion also predispose to impotence and unexplained sterility. Adequate rest and a change of environment, away from pressures, responsibility and social and family commitments are important first steps. A restful and relaxing holiday in natural surroundings is highly recommended for the marriage partners.
- Where psychological inhibitions are a factor in impotency, alcohol can be consumed by both partners in conjunction with sexual activity.

Prostatic Disease

In males, urinary incontinence is a common problem in middle and old age. It occurs as the prostate gland hypertrophies (increases in size) later in life. This results in pain and tenderness in the fork of the thighs and painful urination. Although the following factors contribute to the problem: sexual excesses, weakness of the muscles, impurities in the bloodstream, taking of strong cathartics and improper diet, medical scientists have not been able to determine the exact underlying cause, and many researchers regard a degree of prostatic enlargement to be a normal accompaniment of old age in the male body. Another important prostatic condition is inflammation or infection in the prostate, called prostatitis.

The yogic point of view

According to yogic physiology, prostatic disease occurs as a long-term effect of excessive and imbalanced secretions of the male hormones such as testosterone. Where the pituitary hormones responsible for reproductive and sexual behaviour have been released in excessive and uncontrolled quantities during the earlier decades of active sexual life, the end result may be chronic infection or the uncontrolled and excessive growth of the gland, until it ultimately encroaches inwards upon the urethral passageway which passes through its lobes. As a result, the flow of urine is gradually and progressively obstructed.

214

Although the process of prostatic hypertrophy is usually recognized and diagnosed in middle or old age, it is actually the end result of a long-term process which has its origins in the earlier years of reproductive life. Unless the male sexual metabolism is balanced and controlled during these early years, the influence of testosterone becomes wayward and excessive later on. Overgrowth of the prostate, resulting in loss of urinary continence, is one effect; prostatic cancer may be another.

Further problems

With prostatic hypertrophy, the urge to pass urine becomes more frequent, but can only be satisfied by active straining. In spite of straining to empty the bladder, the result is that only a small amount of urine can dribble through the obstructed urethra. No sooner is this accomplished than the urge recurs; this also goes on at night. Thus the passage of urine becomes a constant and time-consuming preoccupation and the sufferer's movements and lifestyle are limited as he needs to be always in close proximity to a toilet.

Since the bladder can no longer be completely emptied, a stagnant pool of urine starts to build up behind the gland. This can become infected, leading to further irritation and difficulty requiring medical treatment.

Medical management

Surgical procedure for prostatic hypertrophy is known as 'transurethral resection'. It is performed very commonly today in elderly people. The passage through the gland is widened by introducing a fine surgical knife via the penis, so that both urine and semen can flow freely. This surgical procedure is most successful in those older men who find yogic practices impossible because of their age or general debility. However, younger or more active men who are considering surgery are recommended to undertake yogic training for their disorder and then review their state after a few months.

Holistic management of enlarged prostate
There is very good evidence that prostate enlargement can be stopped and even reversed through the use of zinc, adequate amounts of fish oil extract EPA/DHA, selenium, vitamin D3, E and C and lycopene (best source is tomato paste; use 1 teaspoon daily).

Yogic management of prostatic disease
Prostatic hypertrophy can be managed by yogic practices which systematically control the wayward endocrine secretions, shrinking the prostate gland and restoring proper urinary control, especially in the early stages of the disorder. It is often difficult for an elderly man to follow a full and energetic program of asanas, pranayama, shatkarmas and meditation, though we know of some cases of prostatic hypertrophy relieved by pawanmuktasana alone. Middle-aged men who follow the program will obtain good results, while young men who suffer from deep-seated prostatic infections should follow the program assiduously and reduce their sexual activity as much as possible until the disease has been cured.

1. *Surya namaskara*: Should be performed at sunrise, to capacity, building up to twelve rounds or more. It is a very important pranic regenerator.
2. *Asana*: Commence an asana program with the pawanmuktasana and vajrasana series. Later on the following asanas can be adopted gradually, according to one's capacity: trikonasana, ardha padma paschimottanasana, gatyatmak paschimottanasana, shashank bhujangasana, shalabhasana, sarvangasana, druta halasana, chakrasana, dwi pada kandharasana, ushtrasana, matsyasana, tolangulasana, ardha matsyendrasana, bhramacharyasana, vashishthasana, dhanurakarshanasana, pada angushthasana, mayurasana, veerasana, bhadrasana. Sit in vajrasana whenever possible.
3. *Pranayama*: Bhastrika to capacity, in combination with inner retention, moola bandha and jalandhara bandha

216

are recommended to restore energy. Nadi shodhana up to stage 4 should be performed over a six month period. Surya bheda should be practised once or twice a day, up to ten rounds.

4. *Mudra and bandha*: Moola bandha and vajroli mudra twenty-five times daily. Maha mudra and maha bheda mudra up to seven times daily.

5. *Shatkarma*: Neti and kunjal should be practised daily and laghoo shankhaprakshalana once a week.

6. *Relaxation*: Yoga nidra should be practised each after-noon and abdominal breath awareness in shavasana should be practised before sleep.

7. *Diet*: A light diet free of meat and excessive spices and oils is highly recommended. This conserves energy, enabling it to be redirected for healing purposes. Overeating should be avoided and the evening meal should be taken around sunset. Tea and coffee in excess are harmful, and alcohol and tobacco should be discontinued. Drink plenty of water.

8. *Fasting*: One day per week of fasting or missing the evening meal every few days is highly recommended.

9. *Amaroli*: Can be commenced if the protein content of the diet has been reduced.

10. *Rest*: Adequate rest is essential. A lifestyle based on social activity and late nights should be suspended, at least for some months. If possible, staying in an ashram during this period is highly recommended.

Hernia

Hernia is the protrusion of any internal organ through an abnormal opening anywhere in the body. By far the most common forms of hernia are those which occur through sites of natural weakness in the lower muscular wall of the abdomen through which a portion or loop of the intestine may find its way under certain conditions.

Types of hernia

Hernia occurs in both sexes and is a common disorder, affecting more than two percent (one in fifty) of British men. Hernias are classified according to where they occur.

- *Inguinal hernia* is the most common, accounting for over seventy percent of all external hernias. It is twenty times more common in men than women and occurs when a part of the abdominal contents pushes into the inguinal canal. This is a narrow passage in the groin through which the testis descends into the scrotum before birth. The contents of the hernia may pass down into the scrotum which becomes quite large. This form of hernia may be difficult to distinguish from an independent swelling of the testis or scrotum such as hydrocele, and a medical examination is always advised in order to accurately diagnose the scrotal swelling.

- *Femoral hernia* is the next most common type accounting for seventeen percent of all hernias and usually occurs in women. Here the abdominal contents move into the front of the thigh through an opening which carries the femoral artery into the leg. This artery is the major supplier of blood to the leg.

- *Umbilical hernia* is the third most common type, accounting for eight percent of all hernias. Here the hernial sac bulges out through the umbilicus (navel) where a natural weakness in the abdominal muscles exists. This form of hernia usually appears at birth or in infancy, but may also occur in an obese and weak abdomen in middle age.

Hernias are also classified according to whether they are reducible or irreducible.

- A *reducible hernia* is one where the protruding sac can be pushed back inside the abdomen. Frequently the hernia reduces itself whenever the patient lies down, but re-emerges again when he stands up. However, some especially large hernias have to be pushed back. Most hernias belong to this group and can often be benefited by a specific set of yogic asanas learned under careful guidance.

- An *irreducible hernia* is a life-threatening situation and a medical emergency. This occurs when the abdominal contents become caught in the hernia and cannot be pushed back. Such a situation can lead to strangulation, gangrene of the parts in the hernia and even death. Therefore, if this does occur, even if there is no pain one should go immediately to a hospital.

Causes of hernia

A number of factors act alone or in combination to weaken the abdominal muscles. In the first place there may be a developmental defect or a congenital weakness of the abdominal muscles or ligaments, so that a hernia occurs soon after birth. A powerful, sudden, muscular effort such as occurs while lifting a heavy weight without care, may tear muscles and ligaments to produce a hernia and this is the usual cause of hernia in a young man or woman.

Any condition where the intra-abdominal pressure is raised may contribute to a hernia, for example, a smoker's cough continuing for months or years, straining to pass urine which is obstructed by an enlarged prostate, and constipation, accompanied by straining at defecation. In constipation there is generally weakening and dissipation of apana vayu (the aspect of prana responsible for downward propulsion and expulsion of wastes from the body), which necessitates straining. These are major causes of hernia in middle age.

Obesity and habitual overeating, which cause the abdominal wall to be overstretched and the intestines to be overstuffed, cause a raised pressure in the abdomen. Another closely related factor is flabbiness of the abdominal muscles due to lack of exercise, and general sedentary living. As a result of this lifestyle the muscles and skin of the abdomen become loose and flabby. As the abdominal wall loses tone, the abdominal organs begin to sag and the whole abdomen starts to protrude markedly. This is termed *visceroptosis*.

Pregnancy and childbirth also increase abdominal pressure, and frequently contribute to development of hernia in women. A carefully guided yoga program in the periods before, during and after pregnancy will prevent this complication.

Management of hernia

The management of hernia depends on its nature and severity. Yogic practices are the best for preventing herniation, and are often curative for hernias that occur due to weak abdominal muscles and overburdened intestines, especially in newly developing hernias. Most hernias will benefit from a few months of persistent practise of specific asanas, combined with modifications in diet and lifestyle. However, surgical correction of hernia is often successful and is recommended in longstanding hernias, in cases where there is a risk of obstruction or strangulation, or if the hernia has developed to large and unmanageable proportions.

After surgical correction of a hernia, asanas can be adopted under careful guidance and after allowing adequate time for initial healing and recovery. This will ensure that the ultimate outcome of the operation is a positive one. Four to eight weeks after the operation, simple asanas like the pawanmuktasana series part 1 should be adopted. No pressure or strain should be applied to the abdominal muscles for the first three months after surgery. After this time, a few of pawanmuktasana part 2, the shakti bandha series and vajrasana may be adopted under strict guidance. Asana which require forward bending at the waist should not be attempted without guidance, and those major asanas which impose a strain upon the abdomen such as bhujangasana, dhanurasana and shalabhasana should be avoided.

Yoga program for prevention and management of hernia

Precautionary note: No asanas should be practised while a hernia remains in an unreduced state. Any hernia should first be replaced inside the abdomen by expert manipulation.

1. *Asana*: Pawanmuktasana 1 & 2, especially naukasana, ardha titali asana and poorna titali asana. Halasana, pashinee mudra, sarvangasana, matsyasana, vajrasana, shashankasana, marjari-asana, ushtrasana, yoga mudra, vipareeta karani asana, supta vajrasana.
2. *Pranayama*: Bhramari pranayama, mild bhastrika, with antar kumbhaka, jalandhara and moola bandha, and bahir kumbhaka with uddiyana bandha.
3. *Mudra and bandha*: Ashwini mudra, vajroli mudra, moola bandha, agnisar kriya.
4. *Shatkarma*: Jala neti. Laghoo shankhaprakshalana once per week.
5. *Relaxation*: Yoga nidra.

Further recommendations

• Management of hernia involves restoration of proper digestion, correction of constipation and balance of the apana vayu.

- Hernia sufferers should not lift heavy weights. Sneezing, coughing, difficulty while passing urine and stools must be overcome if a hernia is not to recur.
- A light natural vegetarian diet is recommended, with adequate bulk to avoid constipation. Dietary moderation is essential. Never take so much food that stretching of the abdomen and therefore raised abdominal pressure occurs.
- If aggravation of the symptoms of hernia occurs mild fasting is recommended, especially the taking of one meal less per day. This usually makes the condition manageable again.

Hydrocele

Hydrocele is a collection of clear, serous fluid in the tunic or lining of one or both testes in the male. It may be congenital in male infants, but the commonest type in India occurs in adults, where long-term swelling of the testis and spermatic cord is thought to follow repeated acute bouts of infection of the testis and spermatic cord (epididymoorchitis). Hydrocele may develop rapidly or gradually and may be large or small. The disorder occurs in men of all ages, but its onset is frequently in youth. If it is inadequately managed, there may be progressive worsening of the condition as age advances.

Sufferers usually give a history of fluid retention (oedema) in one or both testes, associated with inflammation, swelling and pain of the spermatic cord in the groin. Each bout is associated with some accumulation of fluid about the testis, which finally becomes hard. Gradually the testis becomes enlarged. In cases of recurrent attacks extending over years, where each attack has been inadequately managed, the hydrocele never reducing or reversing itself, it becomes hard and indurated and may become abnormally large.

The cause of hydrocele

Medical scientists recognize that hydrocele may occur due to congenital weakness, traumatic injury or overstraining, while in the tropics hydrocele is commonly due to *filariasis*, an infection due to the roundworm (filaria sanguinis hominis) which is transmitted by a mosquito (culex fatiguans) to the human subject.

Once in the human body, the adult female worm finds its way selectively into the lymphatic circulation and the lymph nodes (especially the inguinal nodes in the groin). There it attains sexual maturity over a period of six to eighteen months, and produces vast numbers of microfilaria. Up to fifty million of these may be circulating in the bloodstream at one time. The earliest symptoms develop six or more months after the initial infection when these regional lymph nodes and the lymph vessels draining the limbs and external genitalia become hot, red painful and tender (lymphadenitis). There are recurrent bouts of fever. Bouts of these symptoms continue to recur intermittently, until irreversible damage to the lymphatic drainage system occurs. The legs or scrotum can become enormous and grotesque as the disease continues.

The vajra nadi

According to yogic science, the failure of lymphatic circulation in the lower extremities is a disorder of the vajra nadi, the flow of prana between the brain and the reproductive organs. Medical science has been unable to directly correlate the presence of filarial infection with the occurrence of hydrocele, and in most cases of hydrocele attributed to filarial infection, no microfilaria are detected in nocturnal blood samples, nor is a past history of filariasis obtained from the sufferer. On the other hand, those whose blood shows a very high microfilaria count often have no symptoms whatsoever.

The most likely explanation is a combination of yogic and medical viewpoints. It appears that excessive heating in the reproductive system, perhaps associated with sexual repression, leads to the cyclical vitiation and degeneration of semen within the spermatic cords. These wastes are drained into the pelvic lymphatic nodes where they selectively attract the filarial parasites to leave the blood circulation and nest in the pelvic lymphatics.

Stasis of seminal fluid in the spermatic cord is the forerunner of stagnation of lymphatic fluid, inflammation and infection of the cord (epididymoorchitis), which leads to swelling (oedema) of the scrotum and ultimately hydrocele. Yoga recognizes that it is a disturbance in the sexual metabolism associated with vajra nadi which is the fundamental problem in this disorder, enabling the opportunistic filaria to manifest symptoms of lymphatic infection.

Treatment of hydrocele

Where filariasis is suspected, the drug Diethyl carbamazine (DEC) often proves effective in the short-term eradication of the symptoms of acute infection. However, the drug is of marginal success in preventing recurrences. Clearly the elimination of the cause requires a deeper yogic understanding of its aetiology and character.

The cycle of build-up and breakdown of semen has to be influenced by yogic techniques, because this is the source of the lymphatic fluid which is becoming infected. The solution is not to increase the release of semen from the body. This is a very short-term measure which only results in increased formation of sperm and activation of the cycle. Rather yoga attempts to influence the psycho-emotional processes responsible for reproductive and sexual metabolism. This offers the prospect of a cure in the early stages, and can be accomplished by a combination of yoga techniques.

In chronic cases, where a permanent hydrocele has developed, surgical drainage is effective; however, this is usually a temporary measure as the fluid reaccumulates rapidly. Surgical intervention should be followed by a daily yoga program to prevent a recurrence of the disorder. Yoga practices can gradually and permanently reduce hydrocele.

Yogic management of hydrocele

These practices will stimulate lymphatic drainage and remove stasis of lymph in the pelvis and lower limbs.

However, they should not be adopted until the acute illness has subsided.

1. *Surya namaskara*: To capacity.
2. *Asana*: Pawanmuktasana part 1, trikonasana, saithalyasana, gomukhasana, sarvangasana, halasana, matsyasana, paschimottanasana, brahmacharyasana, ardha matsyendrasana, vatayanasana, garudasana, sirshasana, tadasana.
3. *Pranayama*: Nadi shodhana, surya bheda, and bhastrika with antar kumbhaka, jalandhara and moola bandhas, and bahir kumbhaka with uddiyana bandha. Practise pranayama in padmasana.
4. *Mudra and bandha*: Vipareeta karani mudra, pashinee mudra and yoga mudra. Practise ashwini mudra, vajroli mudra and moola bandha twenty-six times each, twice a day, preferably while in the inverted postures.
5. *Shatkarma*: Avoid them unless constipation necessitates laghoo shankhaprakshalana.
6. *Relaxation*: Yoga nidra daily.
7. *Meditation*: Antar mouna each night. Try to witness the action of vajra nadi. If this prana can be controlled at its source in the brain, the root cause of the disease has been grasped.
8. *Diet*: Restrict salt intake and avoid heavy foods, rice and watery vegetables.

Further recommendations

- The acute bout of epididymoorchitis, testicular swelling and fever, should be managed by complete bed rest. After acute inflammation subsides (usually one week or more), bed rest should continue. Return to normal life gradually, avoiding strain, especially lifting.
- Standing and walking should be restricted. When standing, the scrotum should be supported by suitable underwear.
- Dry heat fomentation of the scrotum with hot, dry cloth or wild tobacco leaf is useful in reducing swelling and inflammation.

- Whenever going to the toilet, either to pass urine or empty the bowels, grasp the neck of the scrotum firmly and push the testes down to the bottom of the scrotum. Hold for ten seconds, then repeat the procedure three times. This process promotes lymph drainage in the spermatic cords and helps to remove blockage and obstruction. It frequently proves effective in shortening the acute bout and reversing chronic hydrocele.
- Recognition of seminal discharge as a natural function in a healthy male body is an important step. Two nocturnal emissions a month is considered healthy and normal. The problem of hydrocele has been known to disappear after marriage.
- Establish a yogic lifestyle. Do not depend on social life, cinema, etc., for excitement and relaxation. Attain fulfilment through meditation and karma yoga. Develop the mind and the heart through yoga.

Miscellaneous
Disorders

The Skin in
Health and Disease

The skin which covers the human body is a unique and complex living structure. Its outermost cell layers are dead and are continually flaking from the body, yet it is through them that the aura of vitality and good health is reflected to the world like a mirror. Similarly, it is only our skin which upholds the engrossing illusion of our existence – that we are individuals separate from one another. Consciousness is one and universal. The individual mind is an illusion upheld solely by our perception of physical separation. My skin forms the barrier which I believe is the end of me and your skin does the same for you. Physiologically speaking that barrier is nothing but a few layers of flaking, already dead epithelial cells.

The skin is the medium for the sense of touch. It is absolutely essential for many of the most transcendental sensual experiences, both pleasurable and painful. Life without each of the other senses can at least be contemplated, but can you imagine the possibility of having no feeling or touch experience? Touch is the medium through which many emotions, energies and human feelings are communicated. Apart from the subtle aspects of the sense of hearing, we could say that touch is surely the most expressive of the sense modalities.

It is said that beauty is but skin deep. Our physical differences and personal characteristics are very much the attributes of the skin. The skin is an index of good health. A healthy person or yogi is radiant and has a glowing complexion, while a sick person is pale and devoid of prana.

Medical students learn that medical examination commences simply by looking at the patient and assessing his complexion and general demeanor. In light skinned races, diagnosis can frequently be made upon the basis of skin appearance alone. Liver and blood diseases are reflected in a jaundiced skin, pallor reflects shock, anaemia or blood loss, a blue countenance, termed cyanosis, occurs in heart failure and respiratory defects, a red face occurs in valvular heart disease and alcoholism, and a wan, sallow or grey complexion often accompanies kidney disease or cancer.

The skin is an organ
In considering the skin in health and disease, the first point is to realize that the skin is a distinct body organ. An organ is defined as a group of cells clustered together in order to fulfil a specific physiological function. Secondly, the health of the skin cannot be considered in isolation from the rest of the body. Healthy skin is intimately related to diet, the state of the digestive processes, the liver and bloodstream.

The restoration of skin health through yoga therapy is often directed primarily at influencing the digestive and circulatory functions. This is because skin eruptions so commonly reflect a more widespread eliminative, circulatory or metabolic problem, which must first be corrected if skin health is to be restored. It is not sufficient to merely suppress skin diseases with drugs and creams which give only temporary relief but no lasting cure.

The structure of the skin
Under the microscope, the skin is seen to be composed of distinct layers. The outer epidermis, up to thirty cell layers thick, is constantly being shed from the body surface and is replaced by new cell layers arising from the inner layer or dermis. It is also responsible for pigmentation or skin colour.

Beneath the dermis lies the subcutaneous tissue and insulating fat, containing the sweat glands and ducts, hair follicles and sebaceous glands, and the sensory nerve endings or bulbs (Pacinian corpuscles) which relay sensations of touch and pressure to the central nervous system via the sensory cutaneous nerves. Also within this subcutaneous layer lie the tiny blood vessels, arteries, veins and capillaries responsible for supplying the skin cells and glands with oxygen and fuel, and also for carrying away their wastes. The skin, unlike the cells of deeper tissues, also receives nutrients and expels wastes directly to the outside environment and atmosphere via the process of sweating.

The function of the skin

- *Protection*: The skin forms a wonderful protective barrier for the body. A thin layer of natural oil secreted from the skin pores prevents water damage. Weight bearing areas of the body, such as the soles and palms, are thicker and continual pressure or friction can result in calluses.
- *Insulation-heating*: The skin possesses several adaptive mechanisms which enable it to conserve heat in cold climates and yield heat to cool the body in hot conditions, preserving the core body temperature (98.4F or 36.9C). Sweating cools by allowing large amounts of body water to evaporate from the skin surface on a hot day. The small skin arteries possess the ability to dilate in hot conditions or turbulent emotional states, so that blood is drawn towards the skin in order to cool it. The opposite occurs in cold weather.
- *Elimination*: The skin is a major eliminative organ of the body, along with the intestines, the kidneys and the lungs. Water, salt and wastes leave the body through the skin. This is why a person whose body is toxic and unhealthy or whose diet is heavy and impure has an offensive smelling odour, while a healthy person has an inoffensive odour. Many skin rashes, eruptions and diseases are actually attempts by the body to eliminate toxic wastes, which

cannot be expelled in other ways. These occur especially where the bowels are chronically constipated or the kidneys are failing to effectively filter the blood so that wastes begin to build up, clogging the efficient operation of the cells and tissues. The suppression of skin rashes and infection with topical or systemic antibiotics or steroid drugs is often unsuccessful because this aspect of the disease is not well understood. The rash frequently reappears soon after these drugs are discontinued. This is often the stimulus to further suppress it with even greater force. Ultimately, the cause of the rash may be successfully suppressed only to reaccumulate in some other tissue not readily visible to the eye, such as the colon where an abcess, a tumour and perhaps a cancer ultimately develops. This is why skin eruptions are best allowed to run their course if it is possible, while ensuring the best possible conditions for elimination and cure.

• *Absorption*: The skin also plays an important part in absorption. The sun's rays are absorbed and initiate biochemical reactions which produce both skin pigment (melanin) and vitamin D. For this same reason, great care should be taken in dealing with industrial chemicals, fertilizers, fruit sprays, dyes, etc., as many find their way directly into the body when they come into contact with the skin surface. For example, workers in margarine factories where alkaline dyes were used to artificially colour the product were found to develop a high percentage of bladder cancers. Subsequent studies revealed that this chemical dye enters the skin pores and becomes concentrated in the bladder, where it induces cancerous changes in the lining cells.

A medical classification of skin diseases

We have classified skin diseases into the following six categories.

Hypersensitivity or allergy to drugs, chemicals, etc: This type of skin eruption is very common when people are prescribed powerful drugs for common ailments which are often better managed without them. The number and severity of side effects of modern drugs is not well publicized, but every doctor is well aware that the skin, blood, liver, kidneys and digestive system are very commonly injured as a side effect of drug therapy. Such diseases are termed iatrogenic, produced as a side effect of drug therapy for another symptom, and they present a major problem for doctors today. Treatment of an iatrogenic skin rash is to discontinue the offending drug and then purify the body of drug residues through a program of fasting, asana, pranayama and shatkarmas.

Psychosomatic skin disease: The skin is an extremely sensitive mirror of the mind, and skin diseases, rashes and itches such as neurodermatitis often manifest in tense, anxious and sensitive persons. An itch is often a way of expressing the mental tensions arising from personal conflicts. It is recognized in statements such as: "What's biting you?" or "He really gets under my skin." These rashes come and go in response to altering psychic, emotional and personal stresses in life in some temperaments.

Antar mouna, witnessing the itching sensation and the underlying mental tensions without resorting to the unconscious scratching response, is the fundamental step in management of neurodermatitis. Once scratching is resisted and relaxation established, the rash soon disappears. Asana, pranayama and yoga nidra work on the underlying mental and emotional tensions. The hatha yoga shatkarmas – neti, kunjal and shankhaprakshalana – are prescribed to clean the digestive system and purify the nadis (psychic energy flows) in which blockage and obstruction to the pranic flow is occurring.

Contact dermatitis: Many chemical agents cause irritation and eruptions, particularly after prolonged exposure. This is especially so with cosmetics, body lotions, underarm deodorants, hair sprays, insect repellents, dish washing liquids and industrial chemicals. When the offending agent is determined and its use discontinued, the rash also disappears.

235

Skin infections: Skin infections are caused by various micro-organisms, including viruses, bacteria and fungi which live and multiply upon the skin surface. Certain viruses and bacteria do grow naturally on a normal healthy skin, but when the body metabolism becomes unbalanced and the level of vitality drops or wastes accumulate throughout the system, then pathogenic (disease-producing) organisms which find these conditions more favourable begin to multiply rapidly and skin infections result. A wide variety of specific drugs are used for treatment, including antibiotics, steroid creams and anti-fungal agents, either topically or by mouth, and these will provide rapid symptomatic relief. However, skin infections commonly recur because the fundamental cause has not been recognized and the underlying imbalance remains uncorrected. Skin infections can be broadly classified as follows:

- *Viral infections*: 'Shingles' is a very painful skin condition in which vesicles appear in bands on the skin surface caused by the herpes zoster virus. In yogic terminology this occurs because of deficiency or blockage in the flow of prana along the cutaneous nerves. This is usually found in the thoracolumbar nerve roots associated with anahata chakra. As a result, a painful band-like rash appears on the ribcage or chest wall.

  'Cold sores', due to infection by the herpes simplex virus, are another example. Weeping sores appears around the lips and nose during and after a cold, flu or other respiratory infections. They subsequently disappear soon after the body overcomes the primary infection, but will almost inevitably reappear when another cold manifests itself. Cold sores go on appearing and reappearing when the body's levels of resistance and vitality are reduced. This tendency can be overcome by the hatha yoga shat-karmas, surya namaskara and pranayama.

- *Bacterial infections*: These include boils, impetigo and cellulitis and are characterized by the production of pus. Pus is usually a thick, yellowish liquid waste and consists of bacteria and dead white blood cells. Bacterial infections signify stagnation of energy in the skin, impurities in the blood from putrefaction in the digestive system, and improper diet. The body fills with toxic waste matter and is in a low state of resistance. Bacterial infections are best allowed to run their course, but the entire intestine should be washed by shankhaprakshalana to remove constipation and insure effective elimination via the bowels. Boils may also be caused by internal, mental or emotional conflict and confusion.

- *Fungal infections*: These manifest as a moist itching rash and are especially common in the wet, moist and warm areas of the body, for example, between the toes and in the groin. Fungi gain access via the skin's protective barrier when conditions are favourable, for example, when there is an excess of acidity in the body. Acidity is a waste product from cell metabolism and an excess reflects underlying imbalance. They are best managed by internal purification through shankhaprakshalana which will remove excess acidic wastes.

Fungal rashes are notoriously difficult to eradicate permanently by conventional therapy alone. They recur for as long as the underlying imbalance remains uncorrected. They are worsened by synthetic underwear and socks. Like many skin eruptions they are best left clean and dry, open to the sunlight and air, rather than covered up with bandages and dressings.

- *Scabies*: This is an infestation by small mites which burrow within the skin and lay their eggs there, causing intense itching, especially in the wrists, arms and finger webs. The remedy is rubbing the body with benzoyl benzoate oil, followed by boiling all clothing and bedding.

Psoriasis: This unsightly recurrent skin disorder is the cutaneous manifestation of a more deep-set psychophysiological disturbance. An improper, devitalized diet high in carbohydrates, faulty utilization of fats and excess cholesterol in the skin and blood are also contributing factors. No lasting cure for psoriasis exists in medical science, but yogic practices frequently enable an earnest individual to realize and evolve beyond the root cause of this disease. Amaroli should be practised in conjunction with yogic sadhanas, including inverted asana. Expose the affected areas to direct sunlight every day, and try to bathe these areas in salty seawater as often as possible.

Skin cancer: This usually occurs on the face or forearms of fair skinned persons following many years of exposure to direct sunlight in a tropical country. The skin should be shielded by a suitable lotion before exposure and a wide brimmed hat should be worn. The practice of amaroli (massage with three to seven day old urine) in conjunction with dietary modification and pranayama frequently proves successful in its prevention and cure.

Holistic management of chronic skin disorders

It is a well-known truism amongst holistic therapists that the skin is a mirror of digestive health. Diseases such as eczema, dermatitis, psoriasis or urticaria are often found to be related to significant digestive problems, food intolerances and/or parasites in the gut. Chronic itch, without a skin rash, is another extremely annoying condition, which is most commonly caused by liver toxicity. When these issues are methodically identified and treated, the skin problems improve dramatically.

General yogic program for skin health

Specific modification in individual cases may be necessary under skilled guidance.

1. *Surya namaskara*: To the point of total body sweating, while facing the newly rising sun. The sweat should be allowed to dry on the body while resting in shavasana.
2. *Pranayama*: Bhastrika and nadi shodhana pranayama should be practised each morning. Antar and bahir kumbhaka and maha bandha (jalandhara, uddiyana and moola) may be integrated into the pranayama practice.

238

3. *Shatkarma*: Neti, kunjal and laghoo shankhaprakshalana should be performed daily. Poorna shankaprakshalana should be undertaken in an ashram environment, preferably at the commencement of therapy.
4. *Relaxation*: Yoga nidra daily.
5. *Diet*: A light vegetarian diet, rich in alkaline foods (juices, fruit and vegetables). Oil, sweets, refined, fried and spicy food should be avoided and salt and dairy foods restricted. At the commencement of treatment, a raw food diet should be followed for at least five days. Then, for a month, either lunch or the evening meal can be missed.

Further recommendations
- Cold bath and skin rub each morning.
- Sparing use of soap and cosmetics.
- Skin rashes should be kept clean and dry as far as possible and open to the sun and air. The area should be washed free of debris once a day with a mild non-irritant soap, and dried carefully.
- Avoid constipation and keep the digestive system clean.
- Drink plenty of water.
- Amaroli, application of fresh midstream urine, is highly effective in eliminating acute skin rashes. However, the diet should be pure. Urine therapy can also be used in chronic skin diseases such as leucoderma and psoriasis. See *Amaroli*, published by Yoga Publications Trust.

Varicose Veins

Many people complain of a tired, heavy, aching feeling in their legs by the end of the day, a result of inefficient functioning of dilated, lengthened, tortuous varicose veins. This easily recognizable condition only occurs in humans and is related to the special circulatory stresses involved in maintaining an upright posture.

Yoga therapy brings relief to sufferers of this condition and aids in correcting and restoring damaged veins to their former condition. This is especially true of early cases where damage is not yet severe.

The condition is characteristic of middle and old age, but can occur at any time following damage to the muscles and veins of the legs. It can be a result of an hereditary tendency, occurring in families from generation to generation, and frequently accompanies pregnancy. It is an occupational hazard for people who spend long periods of time on their feet, such as machine operators, process workers, traffic policemen, barbers, counter workers, cashiers and tellers.

How do varicose veins develop? To answer this question we must first consider the structure and functioning of the venous return system from the extremities back to the heart. In the average adult body, the column of venous blood must flow at least four feet uphill against gravity, in order to enter the heart. This is quite an engineering feat which nature has accomplished through a system of one-way flow valves lying along the leg veins. The pumping action is established as the muscles of the thighs and calves contract with walking. These repeated contractions squeeze the blood upward along the veins towards the heart. The one-way valves within the veins serve to break up the column of blood and prevent it from flowing back down towards the feet.

It is also necessary to understand a little more about the network of veins draining each leg of blood. There are two systems of veins in the legs – the 'superficial' (flowing just beneath the skin) and the 'deep' (flowing within the muscle of the leg and thigh). The superficial system enters the deep system in two places – in the groin and behind the knee. In addition there are a number of perforating veins along the leg and thigh interconnecting the two systems. Varicose veins develop where the two systems are connected to each other. Normally, blood in the superficial system flows into the deep system, the junctions between the two being protected by one-way valves which prevent any backflow from deep to superficial. Now consider what happens when standing straight and erect. The muscle pump is inactive and the whole weight of the column of blood, exerting pressure up to 90mm Hg, is bearing down upon the valves. A varicose vein can occur in three interrelated ways:

1. A valve becomes incompetent, allowing a high pressure leakage of blood back into the superficial system, distending the superficial vein. Over a period of time the engorged superficial vein becomes enlarged and tortuous.

2. An obstruction of the venous return to the heart, higher up in the abdomen, causes an excessive back pressure in the veins, distending them and forcing the valves to open and become incompetent from above. This occurs classically in pregnancy, where the growing uterus impinges on the inferior vena cava, the major vein in the abdomen. For this reason, varicose veins commonly accompany pregnancy, but valvular competence is usually re-established after delivery, especially if the mother uses yoga therapy in the postpartum period. Tumours

241

obstructing flow can also cause varicose veins and this is why a medical check-up is necessary before starting yoga.

3. In thrombosis (blockage) within the deep veins of the leg, all blood flows via the superficial system, producing dilation and valvular incompetence. This is an uncommon and very serious cause of varicose veins requiring urgent medical treatment. It is characterized by intense pain on stretching the calf muscles.

The most common complaint of varicose vein sufferers is the fatigue and discomfort by the end of each day. This may be accompanied by sharp, localized pains in the sites of the varicose veins, swelling of the ankles by evening and an itchiness of the skin of the legs. Others find the unsightliness of their varicose veins embarrassing and socially restricting, feeling obliged to keep their veins covered when in public and consequently limiting their activities.

Fortunately, utilizing a combination of common sense, yoga practices and medical science, a satisfactory solution to most varicose vein problems can be found.

Surgical treatment

Surgical removal of varicose vein may be found necessary if the condition is severe or incapacitating. It must be remembered, however, that surgery does not remove the underlying tendency to varicose veins and sometimes previously unaffected veins may become varicosed at a later time. Therefore, those who undergo surgery for their condition should adopt the asana program given to facilitate venous return and avoid the possibility of further operation in the future. There are two main treatments of varicose vein:

1. Injection of sclerosing (adherent) substances are made into the vein to join their walls together and to prevent their further use as a venous return pathway.

2. Ligation and stripping of the long superficial veins of the leg is carried out. This entails tying of the ends of the veins and removing them entirely. A number of small cuts is required for this operation and the blood is left to return

to the heart via the deep venous system. The surgeon must ensure that each individual communicating vein is successfully tied off.

Yoga therapy

Asana are very effective in the treatment of mild to moderate varicose veins, providing relief from symptoms and, in some cases, allowing incompetent valves to regain their efficiency. Many sufferers have reported great improvement in their condition with regular and consistent practise of these asana.

All the inverted asana are most important. They allow the stagnant pooled blood to drain back to the heart, permitting damaged veins to resume more normal dimensions and facilitating valvular competence. Remember to rest in shavasana after any inverted posture.

Sarvangasana (shoulder stand pose) should be adopted for several minutes, morning and evening and whenever the legs feel tired and heavy during the day. Sirshasana (headstand pose), although an excellent practice for the condition, is an advanced posture and should not be attempted by beginners or adopted for long periods of time except under direct supervision.

Asana which stretch the muscles of the legs, toning and developing the muscle pump, should be practised regularly as, in many cases, the problem of varicose veins manifests because the pumping system is inefficient and weak. Where the muscles are small and flabby, greater strain and pressure are applied to the valves.

It is often the case that when the efficiency of the pumping system is improved through the practice of these asana, the signs and the symptoms of the varicose veins disappear. Sumeru asana is excellent for this purpose. The heels must be brought to the floor if possible, stretching the calf muscles to their maximum. Tadasana is especially good for stretching the veins and enhancing the muscle pump. Pada hastasana and paschimottanasana, when correctly performed, bring a positive pressure to bear on the leg muscle. Pada sanchalanasana (cycling) is especially beneficial for the veins and muscle of the thighs. Surya namaskra is a dynamic asana series with profound benefits. A few rounds should be included at the beginning of the morning program.

It is up to the individual to decide which treatment is best suited to his condition, depending on the severity of the case and the individual's motivation to help himself. All degrees of varicose veins will benefit from a combination of the various therapies. Remember, varicose veins do not develop overnight and you should not expect to immediately reverse the condition for it will take some time.

Through practice of these asana you will gain immediate relief from aching legs. Over a period of weeks or months, by developing muscle pump and emptying veins of stagnant blood, surprising results can be obtained, especially where the veins are not too abnormal to begin with. It is worthwhile trying this approach before rushing off to the surgeon.

Further recommendations

Simple measures such as these, in conjunction with yogic practices can afford much relief as well as aiding increased self-awareness within our daily routine.

- Avoid standing unnecessarily for long periods of time. If this is not possible, then keep the muscle pump actively working and moving the blood by walking around or flexing and contracting the leg muscles as much as possible. There is a special way of walking which will bring relief. The heel is brought to the ground first with each step and then the calf muscles are consciously used to lift the heel of the back foot as it comes forward, increasing the spring in the step.
- Keep the legs elevated as much as possible to drain the pooled blood from the veins. If you work at a desk, support the legs horizontally rather than down in the usual position. Similarly, your favourite relaxation place should include a comfortable high footrest.

244

During pregnancy, lying on the side will aid venous return by shifting the pressure off the inferior vena cava in the abdomen. Alternatively, the pregnant woman can relax lying flat on the back, with the feet against the wall or on a support.

- Some people find the application of a firm elastic bandage or an elastic stocking each morning most beneficial, but others find this too cumbersome and restrictive. During sleep and when the limbs are elevated, the veins will drain out. Strapping the limb, not too tightly, from above the point of emergence of the varicose vein downward in a spiralling motion will prevent them from filling up during the day and will assist the muscle pump as the muscles contract against the added pressure of the bandage. During the day the bandage can be released periodically, the leg elevated and massaged, and then the bandage reapplied. At the end of the day the bandage must be removed.

- Massage of the legs is very effective in bringing relief from the ache of varicose veins. Many people maintain that massage is not only a palliative therapy, but has a long-term curative potential as well, if it is carried out with awareness and on a regular basis. Massage is most pleasant and relaxing in the evening when the limbs are tired. The movement should be towards the heart, squeezing and milking the tissues of blood. A book on massage will give details of how to massage in the most effective way. This is especially soothing and effective for varicose veins accompanying pregnancy.

Notes ———